Living with Breast Cancer

A Johns Hopkins Press Health Book

Living with Breast Cancer

The Step-by-Step Guide to Minimizing Side Effects and Maximizing Quality of Life

Jennifer A. Shin, MD, MPH
David P. Ryan, MD
Vicki A. Jackson, MD, MPH
with Michelle D. Seaton

Johns Hopkins University Press • Baltimore

Note to the Reader: This book is not meant to substitute for medical care, and treatment should not be based solely on its contents. Instead, treatment must be developed in a dialogue between the individual and their physician. Our book has been written to help with that dialogue.

   Drug dosage: The author and publisher have made reasonable efforts to determine that the selection of drugs discussed in this text conform to the practices of the general medical community. The medications described do not necessarily have specific approval by the US Food and Drug Administration for use in the diseases for which they are recommended. In view of ongoing research, changes in governmental regulation, and the constant flow of information relating to drug therapy and drug reactions, the reader is urged to check the package insert of each drug for any change in indications and dosage and for warnings and precautions. This is particularly important when the recommended agent is a new and/or infrequently used drug.

© 2022 Jennifer A. Shin, David P. Ryan, and Vicki A. Jackson
All rights reserved. Published 2022
Printed in the United States of America on acid-free paper
9 8 7 6 5 4 3 2 1

Johns Hopkins University Press
2715 North Charles Street
Baltimore, Maryland 21218-4363
www.press.jhu.edu

Library of Congress Cataloging-in-Publication Data
Names: Shin, Jennifer A., 1977– author. | Ryan, David P., 1966– author. |
    Jackson, Vicki A., 1968– author. | Seaton, Michelle D., author.
Title: Living with breast cancer : the step-by-step guide to minimizing
    side effects and maximizing quality of life / Jennifer A. Shin, MD, MPH,
    David P. Ryan, MD, Vicki A. Jackson, MD, MPH, with Michelle D. Seaton.
Identifiers: LCCN 2021055038 | ISBN 9781421444437 (paperback) |
    ISBN 9781421444444 (ebook)
Subjects: LCSH: Breast—Cancer—Popular works. |
    Breast—Cancer—Patients—Care—Popular works. |
    Breast—Cancer—Psychological aspects—Popular works. |
    Breast—Cancer—Patients—Life skills guides.
Classification: LCC RC280.B8 S4935 2022 | DDC 616.99/449—dc23/eng/20211207
LC record available at https://lccn.loc.gov/2021055038

A catalog record for this book is available from the British Library.

Special discounts are available for bulk purchases of this book. For more information, please contact Special Sales at specialsales@jh.edu.

Every cancer specialist has received phone calls from friends of friends who have a breast cancer diagnosis or are in treatment and who have many unanswered questions. These patients have all heard what the doctor said to them in clinic—or thought they did—but afterward they often have trouble making sense of that information. This confusion is completely understandable. There are few things more disorienting than hearing the words, "You have cancer." Every phase of treatment can seem equally disorienting as the person enters a new world filled with tests and scans and jargon. Patients are often at a loss about how to ask the right questions of their oncologists and nurse practitioners about the treatments they undergo. They struggle to talk in detail about their emotions and symptoms in a busy clinical setting.

In 2016, Dave Ryan and I wrote the book *Living with Cancer: A Step-by-Step Guide for Coping Medically and Emotionally with a Serious Diagnosis*. We hoped it would help people with any type of cancer cope with cancer treatments and the possible progression of cancer. It was meant as a sort of field guide to cancer care and we hoped that patients would use it to get their bearings in treatment and better communicate their needs and questions to their medical team.

Living with Cancer sprang from a novel integrated approach to cancer care at the oncology division at Massachusetts General Hospital. Patients with a serious diagnosis are offered the opportunity to meet with both an oncologist and a palliative care specialist. The oncologist can focus on tests and scans and treatments for the cancer, while the palliative care specialist with expertise in symptom management focuses on how you are living with the cancer and the treatments. It's like meeting with an additional practitioner, someone who is focused on how you are really doing both physically and emotionally living in this new cancer world.

That book was the product of more than 10 years of working with many of the same patients, answering their questions while also offering each other our different perspectives on patient care. In that time, we learned that it's not easy to stay oriented in the complex world of cancer treatment. People often need to hear information more than once. They need strategies to help them live fully and take advantage of the days when they feel strongest. And they love hearing about how other patients have dealt with situations similar to theirs. That book was the result of all of that work with our patients. We wanted to create a guide for people to help answer their questions and empower them to ask many more questions of their own medical care team members.

After it was published, we heard from many patients who found the book extremely useful. We also heard from other patients who wanted a book that dealt only with breast cancer, because it's a disease that affects more than 3 million women and thousands of men in the United States. Breast cancer is unique in that very shortly after diagnosis, a person has to learn a new vocabulary that describes their cancer cells. They may need to make decisions about the type of surgery to get and how to cope with a new body. They may also be hearing about various treatments, each with its own side effects. And although the success rate with breast cancer treatments offers a lot of hope, people may find themselves living with uncertainty about the future that lasts long after treatment ends. These are things that a palliative care perspective can help with.

Researchers have long documented the benefits of early integrated palliative care on people with a serious diagnosis, such as metastatic cancer. Quality of life is higher and rates of depression are lower. It reduces the burden of care on family members. It gives individuals the confidence to work with their medical teams to reduce symptoms and side effects of treatment, and it encourages them to live fully regardless of the prognosis. With all of that in mind, we wrote this book to describe how patients can take advantage of the palliative care perspective while in treatment for any stage of breast cancer.

To do this, Dave and I enlisted the help of Dr. Jennifer Shin, who is a palliative care specialist and a breast cancer oncologist with years of experience in both specialties. We also worked again with Michelle Seaton, a medical writer who helped craft our ideas into the book you hold now. Because of privacy concerns, the patient stories you read here are composites based on the many thousands of patients we have treated.

Living with Breast Cancer reflects our understanding that the breast cancer experience is very different today than it was even a few years ago. New treatment options abound, including new targeted therapies, for all types of breast cancer, which means that people who receive anti-cancer therapies often do well for a long time, even if they have metastatic disease. We firmly believe that patients with a breast cancer diagnosis do better and feel better if they have a dedicated resource that helps them to manage the symptoms and side effects of treatment, one that encourages them to think about their goals, about the future, and about their quality of life. Patients feel more empowered when they have someone encouraging them to track and talk about their symptoms, someone who is offering them strategies for maximizing their quality of life. We want this book to be that resource. We want people to concentrate on today, on living the best life they can right now.

Vicki A. Jackson, MD, MPH

ACKNOWLEDGMENTS

The authors wish to thank several colleagues who contributed to this book. Jerry Younger, MD, is a retired breast oncologist from Massachusetts General Hospital (MGH) who reviewed the manuscript in its entirety before publication, providing necessary feedback to the authors. Rachel B. Jimenez, MD, is a radiation oncologist at MGH who provided important feedback on the sections related to radiation therapy. Mark L. Zangardi, PharmD, BCOP, and Jennifer A. Hutchinson, PharmD, BCOP, have both worked as breast oncology clinical pharmacists at MGH. They provided valuable information about breast cancer therapies for the tables in this book.

PART ONE *Making Sense of Your Diagnosis*

CHAPTER ONE

How Am I Going to Get Through This?

Vicki answers first:

I'm sorry that you have to read this book. This is probably the last place you thought you would be, reading a book about dealing with a diagnosis of breast cancer or helping someone you love adjust to this new reality. It can all feel surreal and overwhelming—the diagnosis, the medical jargon, the treatment options, and the need to find specialists who can help you and with whom you feel comfortable. After a preliminary diagnosis, you may have a lot of urgent appointments for tests and further scans, or a biopsy or surgery, while also enduring days of anxious waiting. Throughout all of this it may seem impossible to believe any of the results. You want to shake the world and shout, "This can't be happening!"

It's hard for most medical professionals to fully understand the profound changes that people are asked to go through when they receive a cancer diagnosis. I got a glimpse of this shortly after I became a palliative care doctor. I remember standing in the lobby of a hospital in Boston on the morning of 9/11. We'd gathered there after news of a hijacking had spread, and we watched on TV as the towers collapsed. Like everyone else I kept watching it over and over again because I couldn't grasp what was going on. I saw it, but I couldn't quite believe it. That's when a patient took my arm and said, "That feeling you all have right now—that it's so unreal, that it can't be true. That's what it feels like to be told that you have cancer." I'm so grateful that he said that to me, because I now know that the first thing you have to get your mind around is how to understand that this is happening at all.

Very quickly you have many more things to do as well. You have to build some kind of familiarity with your type of cancer and the obscure names of all the body parts affected by it. You have to learn to listen to an oncologist describing scans and lymph nodes and maybe the relative benefits of surgery, hormonal therapies, or chemotherapy and radiation. You have to figure out how to start a treatment regimen that will come with a long list of possible side effects. You have to find some context for your diagnosis and think about the future, knowing that it's going to be very different from what you had imagined. On top of that, you have to figure out how to keep living your life as normally as possible.

Having worked with thousands of patients who were dealing with a cancer diagnosis, I know that people need help with all of this. And I know that while Internet searches can sometimes be helpful, different websites can offer advice that is conflicting or even confusing. It's relatively easy to search for survival rates and treatment options; it's harder to figure out what these facts have to do with your situation. It's often bewildering to translate those facts into questions to ask your care team at various points in treatment.

That's why Dave and I wrote our first book, *Living with Cancer: A Step-by-Step Guide for Coping Medically and Emotionally with a Serious Diagnosis*. It was a way to help guide cancer patients and their families through the common issues they would face during treatment, no matter what type of cancer they had. We wanted to help people understand what has been said to them in their appointments and during chemotherapy treatments. Dave is a medical oncologist, and I'm a palliative care specialist. Together we've worked with thousands of patients, answering their questions about the likely course and outcome of their disease (prognosis) and treatment options, as well as helping them cope day to day. We have watched people go through this process and helped them get their bearings again. We've helped them feel confident and capable of getting through treatment while living their lives as fully as possible.

Shortly after the book was published, Dave and I started hearing from patients and cancer specialists that they would like to see another book, one that specifically applied this model to the treatment of breast cancer. And it's true that breast cancer diagnosis and treatment is different from other cancers. Many women have been getting mammograms or doing self-exams for years, which means that they may have thought about or worried about this diagnosis for a long time. Breast cancer is a big part of our public awareness, and many patients know several women who have been treated for breast cancer. This doesn't make the diagnosis any less overwhelming. There's so much to learn and understand as you ponder the goals of treatment, the specific surgeries that would be right for you, and what life will be like in treatment. I hope this book will help with all of that. It can be a resource when you come home from a medical appointment and need some context for what your medical team has said to you. It can also help empower you to advocate for yourself to minimize the symptoms and side effects of treatment so that you can live your life fully during treatment.

Shortly after diagnosis, this may seem like an impossible goal, but you can do it. Armed with the right information, you can understand what each specialist is saying to you. You can make this less surreal. You can go on living your life.

Both books grew from the professional relationship that Dave and I formed at Massachusetts General Hospital (Mass General) in Boston. Almost twenty years ago, the hospital created an outpatient palliative care program, designed to give cancer patients the chance to meet regularly with a specialist who works closely with their medical team. This provider acts like a primary care practitioner for their cancer care, going over all of their prescriptions, addressing their side effects, and asking about their emotional health and whether they need additional services to support them or their families.

At that time most oncologists referred patients to palliative care only at the end of life, to help them deal with the unique medical and emotional concerns that arise after anti-cancer treatments have been suspended. Some oncologists didn't understand how their patients would benefit from seeing an additional doctor or nurse practitioner earlier in treatment.

And yet, when I met with patients, I found that I was sometimes the first person to ask them how they were spending their time every day, how they were sleeping, and whether there was anything they wanted to do that they couldn't because of treatment. I also asked them detailed questions about how they were doing in the days after an infusion (intravenous chemotherapy) and went over all of the medications given to treat their symptoms, asking, "Is this working for you?" and "How well is it working?" or "Should we try something else?" Sometimes I found that patients were living with pain or constipation or other side effects that could be minimized with different medications, but they had not wanted to bring them up at the clinic. They wanted to put on a brave face for their oncologist. And that's normal. It's understandable. But my patients discovered that talking about their pain or nausea or anxiety and getting some help could change their lives. They could learn to track their symptoms and go into their appointment with a list and expect the medical team to address all of their concerns.

Some patients didn't know that they could tailor their treatments to minimize the disruption in their work schedules. Others didn't know that they could schedule a chemo holiday—a short break from treatment—to travel or attend a big family event. My hope is that this book will help you take control of your treatment.

The truth is that there is a gap between what traditional cancer care provides and what patients need. I don't blame oncologists for this. Medical oncology is an increasingly complex field. Every year brings more treatment options, new lines of chemotherapy, and new combinations of therapies. Top oncologists are busier than ever, and they have been taught to focus primarily on interventions that will kill cancer cells. It's what they have to do because the stakes are so high. And so much of the burden falls on patients and their family members to understand what's happening to their bodies and their lives.

During the first few years that I worked with cancer patients, there was little coordination between medical oncology and palliative care. Oncologists assumed that palliative care specialists didn't understand the virtues of chemotherapy and how much better patients feel when they have a great response to chemotherapy. And some palliative care specialists worried that oncologists were giving patients regimen after regimen of chemotherapy without paying enough attention to the side effects of treatment or the patient's quality of life. Neither of these assumptions was entirely correct, but they persisted. We had a lot to learn from each other. I had to learn about chemotherapy and how it worked and when it worked best. Oncologists had to learn how palliative care could help patients live better while they were receiving chemotherapy.

Many oncologists were slow to understand how to integrate this kind of care into their clinical practice, but Dave was an early proponent of palliative care. He understood what I was trying to do for patients in the cancer clinic. I hoped that if these two subspecialties could work together, we could create a powerful benefit for patients. We could make cancer treatment much more manageable for them. We could help them better understand a difficult prognosis and live their lives to the fullest while dealing with cancer.

Then Dave and I had a conversation one day that changed everything. It was about 10 years ago, long before he had become the chief of hematology/oncology. At the time, he was a busy and well-respected GI (gastrointestinal) cancer specialist. That day I bumped into Dave in the cancer clinic and told him that I'd just met with one of his patients, a woman named Rebecca who had esophageal cancer. Her scans had come back showing that her cancer had grown through the first line of treatment. I clearly remember asking Dave what chemotherapy he would start her on next. Was he thinking about paclitaxel? He said yes, and I asked whether neuropathy (tingling or numbness in the hands and feet) was one of the common side effects. He said it was. I told him that Rebecca was already dealing with significant neuropathy from her first line of treatment. Was there another option? He later told me that he was stunned by this conversation, in part because Rebecca hadn't told him how much neuropathy she had been experiencing. I'll let him tell his side of the story.

* * *

I remember that conversation with Vicki really well. First, it was surprising to hear a palliative care doctor asking about a specific line of chemotherapy. Second, I was shocked that another doctor knew more about my patient's side effects than I did. I already knew that Vicki worked well with my patients, helping them cope with pain or other issues. Sometimes I would remind a patient about trouble with nausea after an infusion during our last visit and ask for more details, only to have the patient say, "Oh, I talked to Vicki about that. She took care of it." But this conversation about Rebecca's neuropathy had an impact on the regimen I chose for her, and it hinted at a much larger collaboration and how it could improve a patient's care.

It may be surprising to hear that a patient would keep a significant side effect secret from her doctor. After many years of working with palliative care, I've learned that it's actually not unusual for patients to be stoic about their side effects around their oncologists. Some people just want their oncology appointments to focus on treatments. Others don't know that their side effects could be better managed. A few people want to seem strong and capable to their oncologists, or perhaps they downplay unpleasant side effects because they don't want to disappoint their care team. People need help advocating for themselves when it comes to the issues that arise in the cancer setting.

I've learned a lot from Vicki and from her team members about how to better help my patients manage these side effects so they can feel better and more like themselves day to day. I've learned to ask patients how they spend their time and what they want to be doing that they can't because of treatments. I've also learned how to better explain prognosis, and I don't worry if I have to explain these things more than once.

In the past 15 years, outpatient palliative care has become a kind of mission at Mass General, specifically in the cancer clinic. Vicki has since become the chief of the palliative care division, and her team has grown more than 400%. Members of the oncology team, including nurses and nurse practitioners, have come to count on this palliative care perspective. We know that we are providing a singular level of care to patients coping with a difficult diagnosis.

Vicki and her team have been providing palliative care for cancer patients for nearly two decades, and their latest research shows that this perspective can help patients earlier in their disease course. With the right information and encouragement, you can get your arms around this diagnosis. Many patients with an early-stage diagnosis think that they have to be tough and stoic and endure the treatments. But by focusing on your quality of life and your own goals and values, you can do more than that. You can go on living your life fully while in treatment.

Rather than describe the collaboration between palliative care and oncology, we've created a book that will allow you to take advantage of everything that we've learned together and apply it to your breast cancer treatment. Many patients don't yet have access to this kind of team approach, and yet they can benefit from what we know. Nearly every week, we get phone calls from friends of relatives who have a new diagnosis and so many questions. Why did the oncologist tell me this and what does it mean? What do I ask at my next appointment? When will we know if the treatment is working?

Sometimes we get calls from distant friends with parents facing a difficult diagnosis. They ask what to do if the oncologist is recommending chemotherapy but their parent doesn't want it. How can they communicate their parent's wishes to the care team? Very few people have a friend of a friend who practices cancer care at a major teaching hospital. We wanted to tell readers what we tell people on the phone, and we want to talk to readers the same way we would talk to any friend, family member, or patient about the medical issues that arise with this kind of diagnosis.

You won't need to read every chapter of this book. Not every patient has every symptom of cancer, and our hope is that you can turn to whatever chapters you need when you need them. Part One will take you through the initial stages of diagnosis and getting acclimated to treatment. Part Two will help you troubleshoot any symptoms and side effects of treatment. Part Three will walk you through what to expect and what to ask if your cancer continues to advance. Although most people won't need to read the last few chapters especially, we have also included how to deal with end-of-life issues.

In order to write this book, Vicki and I invited one of our colleagues at Mass General, a breast cancer specialist, to help us out. Dr. Jennifer Shin is the perfect coauthor because she is trained as a specialist in breast cancer oncology and is also a trained palliative care provider. She is part of a new generation of oncologists who have been steeped in the palliative care perspective.

Jenn has written the chapters in which the medical oncology perspective is most helpful. Vicki has written the chapters in which she can offer her palliative care expertise on matters such as coping with pain, nausea, weight loss, and other side effects, as well as coping emotionally. I've worked on the chapters in which we talk about progressing cancer, with Jenn's input. It's not important to focus on who has written any individual chapter, though. We want this book to show how this collaboration can give you the widest possible perspective on everything you may encounter in breast cancer treatment, regardless of your specific diagnosis.

Every year brings multiple advances in the field of breast cancer treatment. There are new treatments, including immunotherapy, and targeted therapies and newer lines of chemotherapy. While these treatments may give more patients a much better chance at a cure, they also mean that more cancer patients are living longer with this diagnosis, even when the cancer can't be cured.

I'll let Jenn talk more about her unique perspective on palliative care in breast cancer treatment and how it informs this book.

* * *

I went through specialty training as a palliative care doctor right before my specialty training as an oncologist. This allowed me to see breast cancer care through the lens of a palliative care specialist. I learned to keep a focus on a patient's quality of life and her goals in every phase of treatment. Ultimately I decided to practice both as an oncologist and as a palliative care specialist. So on some days I see my breast cancer patients in the cancer clinic. Other days I report to the palliative care clinic where

I see patients who have other types of cancer or other illnesses. On one occasion, I saw the same patient in both clinics. Let me explain.

A couple of years ago, I met Elizabeth in the breast oncology clinic because she wanted a second opinion. Elizabeth had been diagnosed with an early-stage breast cancer about eight years before. She was treated successfully and was doing great for almost five years when she felt some bothersome pain in her hip. That's when she got the news that her breast cancer had recurred. We talked about hormonal therapy options for her and discussed treatments that might help with her pain and anxiety. Armed with this information, she went back to her oncologist to start treatment. A few months later, I was surprised to see her in my office at the palliative care clinic. She said that she was feeling much better overall and that her tumor was stable, which was great to hear. Elizabeth said she referred herself to palliative care because she wanted to have additional time to focus on her quality of life. She had set specific goals for herself. She wanted to get back to her job as a legal assistant, and she wanted to make sure we were doing everything possible to reduce her pain so that she could function well at work. She also wanted to take vacations with her husband and help plan her daughter's wedding, so we needed to think about strategies to manage her energy levels and reduce her anxiety.

Over the next two years we worked to make sure she was feeling her best so that she could pursue the things that were most important to her. She did attend her daughter's wedding and is now awaiting a first grandchild. Over time she grappled with the decision to retire from her job on her own terms, and not because of the cancer. On a recent visit, we reflected on the past two years and she said to me, "This is what I was hoping for. I wanted to live my life fully while also being treated for cancer."

I also vividly remember my first visit with Charlene six years ago. She was a new mother who had noticed a lump while breastfeeding her 8-month-old daughter. After a mammogram, ultrasound, and biopsy, she was diagnosed with an early-stage breast cancer that had spread to several lymph nodes. Like many women, Charlene had learned of her diagnosis through a phone call from her primary care physician. By the time of our first meeting, she had spent hours online looking up every test she had undergone and looking for stories about women her age with breast cancer. During our first meeting, I don't recall ever seeing her eyes. She had a baseball cap pulled down over her face, and she seemed withdrawn, giving single-word answers to each of my questions. When I asked her about the possibility of doing chemotherapy prior to her surgery, she seemed distracted and overwhelmed.

During our second meeting, she told me that she didn't remember much of what we'd discussed before. We had talked about the fact that her cancer had a high chance of being curable, but she told me that she had trouble making sense of that information. She admitted that she was terrified and that she felt she needed to do as much research as possible in order to make the best decisions for herself and for her family. All of this is normal. I went over everything that we'd talked about before and told her that I could explain it as many times as she needed. Within a few weeks she had begun to manage her anxiety and ask more direct questions about how her chemotherapy would affect the type of surgery she would need. And within a few months, she was fully in the swing of treatment and could share stories about her daughter's early milestones of crawling and sitting up.

Six years later, Charlene still comes in for her annual visits, and I am struck by how vibrant she seems. She laughs as she talks about her kids and her career. It's not that she is a different woman. Actually, she is more like the person she was prior to her diagnosis. The treatments were successful, as we'd all hoped. So, in our visits, we review the results of her yearly mammogram and talk about her general health. Charlene still worries about the possibility that her cancer will come back, but that worry has decreased over time. She is still a patient with a history of breast cancer and has been touched by and changed by the diagnosis and treatment, but she has allowed her life to fill in again, with breast cancer more at the periphery.

That's what I hope this book will offer you—the information that can help you understand your diagnosis and the empowerment to talk to your medical team about the symptoms and side effects of treatment so that you can continue to pursue your life goals. In the weeks after diagnosis, this might seem to be an impossible goal, but I've seen so many patients take up this challenge.

CHAPTER TWO

Setting the Goals for Treatment

Many women are diagnosed with breast cancer after their routine screening mammogram detected something suspicious. Others felt a lump in the breast or armpit or noted skin changes in their breast or nipple. A few people may initially see a doctor because of back pain, headaches, or other symptoms that do not seem to be related to the breast.

If you had an abnormal screening mammogram, or felt a lump, the next step will usually be a mammogram that takes a closer look at the area in question. Doctors call this a diagnostic mammogram. A focused ultrasound of the breast and armpit is sometimes performed at the same time. The ultrasound provides information about whether the lump might actually be a cyst or if the lump is something more solid that might need to be biopsied. Sometimes, a doctor will order a breast MRI (magnetic resonance imaging), particularly if the breast tissue is noted to be very dense. Occasionally, there is only a lump in the armpit and nothing detectable on a mammogram and ultrasound. An MRI can help take a closer look at the breast tissue in these circumstances as well.

If the breast imaging shows something suspicious, a biopsy is usually the next step. For a biopsy, a doctor takes a sample of tissue with a needle. The breast imaging team usually uses the ultrasound, mammogram, or MRI to guide the biopsy needle into the correct spot. This is done while the patient is awake, using a local anesthetic to help with any discomfort. The biopsy itself can be uncomfortable for many patients, and this is often accompanied by the anxiety of the procedure and the fear of hearing what the results might be. Individuals may have some swelling and bruising at and around the biopsy site, which will start to improve in the days after the procedure. This tissue is then sent to the pathologist, who examines it under a microscope to make a diagnosis.

You may have learned of your initial diagnosis while sitting in a primary care provider's office, or even over the phone, and it was probably hard to grasp any of the details about the biopsy after you heard the words, "You have breast cancer." It's often overwhelming to think about finding an oncology team and starting treatment. I (Jenn) always tell new patients that they will likely feel more at ease after our initial meeting. It's reassuring to have a plan in place and to have some idea of what to expect.

In this chapter, I'll walk you through what to expect at your first meeting with a breast cancer oncologist. I'll talk about the kinds of information the oncologist will discuss with you about your cancer and your treatment options, and I hope this will give you ideas about questions to ask and a sense of how your goals and values will play a part in your treatment plan.

Preparing for the First Visit

During your first appointment with an oncologist, you will get a lot of information about your diagnosis and often the treatment plan. This first appointment may feel overwhelming, but it is a kind of road map for the journey ahead. We will review and explain all of the data, instructions, and side effects as many times as you need. And I remind people that they can and should call the clinic with any questions that arise later on. Rest assured that you are going to get to know your team, and they will get to know you, too. I usually say that we are the family you never wanted to have but become really fond of. On that first day, most patients feel that they will never get used to the routine of treatment, but they do. Within a few weeks, they know so much about what a day of treatment looks like that they could walk a friend through the process.

Most people bring a friend or family member to that first visit, in fact. This person can be an extra set of ears. If you have questions, write them down and bring them with you, particularly if you have specific concerns about treatment. Let the doctor know if you have an important event or family milestone coming up. As an oncologist, I also like to know how much information you want to have about your diagnosis and treatment. Some people want to know every detail about possible side effects and tests for many months ahead. Others want to take things week by week. Some want a specific family member to be included in medical decisions. All of this is helpful information so that your medical team can better care for you. Cancer treatments will go after the cancer itself, but your team is here to help you meet your goals and to treat the whole you.

The Initial Visit

A lot is going to happen in your first meeting with an oncologist, and you'll have a better chance of staying oriented if you know what questions the doctor is likely to ask you before talking about your diagnosis, your pathology report, and the recommended treatment. The first half of every initial appointment is really a chance for the oncologist to gather significant information about your medical history. You may have already filled out lots of forms or reviewed this recently with other doctors, so this may seem repetitive. I let people know that although I have thoroughly reviewed the electronic medical record prior to our visit, no one knows your history like you do, and it's helpful to make sure that I have things right. After this initial part of your visit, you will be reviewing lots of details more specific to your cancer and will have a lot of time to ask questions toward the second half of the appointment.

Chief Complaint

This is a fancy term for "what brings you here?" Sometimes doctors will send patients to an oncologist without fully explaining to them that they have cancer. It's helpful for me to know why you think you're in my office. The oncologist may also ask for what's called a "history of present illness," which is a list of what symptoms you may have experienced in the past few weeks and whether you've undergone any tests to reach a diagnosis. You may have been feeling completely well before your visit if your cancer was detected on your yearly mammogram, so you can just report that to your doctor.

Review of Symptoms

The doctor will want to know how you are functioning in daily life. Are you sleeping? Are you in any pain? You may have to answer questions about your anxiety level, your bowels, your eating habits. Are there any activities that you can't engage in because of symptoms? Your doctor may want to help you relieve certain symptoms right away, even before your cancer treatment starts.

Medical History

What are your medical problems, aside from breast cancer? You may have filled out numerous forms detailing a lot of this, but the doctor will want to review them briefly as a way of keeping these details in mind as you both go forward.

Gynecologic History

If you are a woman, your oncologist may ask you how old you were when you began to menstruate. You may be asked the date of your most recent period, or when you went through menopause. You may be asked about how many pregnancies you have had and how old you were when you had your first baby, whether you ever took oral contraceptive pills, and whether you were ever treated with hormone replacement therapy.

Family History

Do you have a family history of breast, ovarian, or any other cancers? If so, which family members and how old were they when they were diagnosed?

Social History

Your doctor may ask where you live, what you do or did for work, and what your family supports are. You will be asked about whether you are currently smoking or previously smoked, how much alcohol you consume, and whether any other recreational drugs are being used.

Medications

Your doctor will want to know your current medications and doses, and if you have a list of them, it's good to bring it to the appointment. Your doctor will also ask whether you have any allergies to medications.

Physical Exam

This is an opportunity for the doctor to look for any signs of the tumor elsewhere in your body. Usually this is brief, and often it's just a formality if we already know what we are going to find from the scans that you have had done. But your doctor wants to get every piece of information available.

Imaging Studies, Possible Labs

The doctor will review the results of any scans you may have had before your appointment. This may include your breast imaging studies, or if more advanced cancer is suspected you may have had CT (computed tomography) scans, bone scans, or other imaging studies. These additional scans are often called "staging scans" because they help us assess your stage at diagnosis. Sometimes labs and imaging studies (beyond breast imaging) are not needed or are checked after your visit, so don't worry if you haven't had these things done.

* * *

All of this should take place in the first half of your appointment. Don't be alarmed if the doctor seems to want to take in all of this information at a brisk pace. Technically, this is a review of available information, but it's a necessary review. Some patients want to skip this part and get directly to the diagnosis and treatment plan. Your best strategy is to let the doctor ask all of these initial questions, answer them succinctly, and then be ready to take notes and ask a lot of questions when the doctor gets to the next part: going over the pathology report on your biopsy, giving you what doctors call the clinical picture. This is when your doctor discusses his or her impression—or diagnosis—and then recommends what kind of treatment would be best.

The Biopsy Report

If you've had a biopsy, the cells taken from your tumor are sent to a pathologist who studies them. There are many key details that the breast biopsy results can tell us about your cancer. This report will answer important questions about the type of cancer cell, the grade of the cells, and the receptor status.

Type

There are several subtypes of breast cancer based on the type of breast tissue affected. For example, the breast contains lobules where breast milk is made and ducts that carry the milk to the nipple. So your cancer may be defined as ductal or lobular. If the tumor cells have invaded other tissues, they are called invasive. About 70% to 80% of breast cancers are invasive ductal carcinomas. Another 10% are invasive lobular carcinomas. The remaining cancers are less common and include mixed ductal/lobular, mucinous, tubular, metaplastic, medullary, and papillary carcinomas.

A note about DCIS: Sometimes, the pathology report will show ductal carcinoma in situ (DCIS). DCIS is a noninvasive cancer, which means that the cancer cells are contained within the breast duct and therefore do not have the ability to spread to other parts of the body, or metastasize. DCIS can be found along with invasive cancer or can be found by itself, without any invasive cancer. When DCIS is found along with invasive cancer, the treatment of the invasive cancer is the focus. The treatment of DCIS when found on its own (stage 0 cancer) is not directly covered in this book.

Grade

I often explain that the grade is how friendly or ugly the tumor cells look under a microscope. Uglier-looking cells tend to divide more aggressively and speed the tumor's growth. A grade 1 tumor usually means the cancer is slower growing, while grade 3 is likely to grow faster. Remember that grade and stage are often confused because they are represented by a number. But you can have a grade 3 tumor that is still stage 1 cancer, which has a high chance of being curable. I will explain how we determine the stage of cancer in another section.

Receptor Status

Receptors are proteins in cells or on the surface of the cell that, when triggered, stimulate cancer cells to grow. The pathologist will test cells from a biopsy for three main receptors—estrogen, progesterone, and something called the human epidermal growth factor type 2 receptor. Doctors refer to the last one as HER2.

If tumor cells contain estrogen receptors (ER), your doctor will say they are ER-positive (or ER+) and if they contain progesterone receptors (PR), they will be PR-positive (or PR+). About 70% of breast cancers contain at least one of these receptors and doctors tend to group them together, calling them hormone receptor–positive cancers. This means that the estrogen in your system is promoting the growth of the tumors. But it also means that your treatment will include anti-estrogen therapies (also known as hormonal or endocrine therapies) that will target these receptors.

About 15% of breast cancers show a lot of HER2 receptors on the surface of the tumor cells, which means that the cells rely on these receptors in order to grow. If your tumor cells are HER2-positive (or HER2+), you may be treated with specific antibodies to block these receptors, usually in addition to chemotherapy. Some cancers that are HER2-positive are also positive for hormone receptors, while others are not. Knowing the receptor status of your tumor is important because it helps your doctor find the best strategies for your treatment.

Some breast cancers don't show any of these receptors and are known as triple-negative cancers. That means that hormone therapies and HER2-directed therapies won't be effective in treating these cancers. If your cancer is triple negative, your best treatment options involve chemotherapy.

Postsurgical Pathology

If you have had breast surgery, the pathology report will also contain information about the tumor as well as the tissue and lymph nodes around it. In some cases, tests will be performed on the cells to look at the activity of tumor genes. You will want to ask your doctor about the information contained in this pathology report. This information helps your doctor determine the stage of your cancer and your treatment plan.

Size

When the tumor in a breast is removed, the pathologist will be able to measure its overall dimensions. In general, the smaller the tumor, the better. Sometimes the surgeon might note other smaller tumors nearby, also called satellite tumors, that are probably part of the same cancer.

Margins

You may have heard that having "clear" or "negative" margins is a good thing. This means that the surgeon removed all of the tumor along with a little bit of healthy tissue around it. If there were no cancer cells detected at the outer edges of this tissue, you have clear margins. If some cancer cells were detected in this tissue, you have positive margins, which means it is possible that there might be cancer still left in the breast, and you may need additional surgery.

Lymph Node Involvement

Sometimes a breast exam reveals small tumors in the armpit. Breast imaging can also reveal enlargement of lymph nodes, suggesting that there may be cancer within them. If your lymph nodes are enlarged, you may also have had a fine needle aspiration or a regular needle biopsy (core biopsy) of your lymph nodes. If any of these showed cancer, the surgeon may have removed additional lymph nodes in the armpit to see if they contain cancer cells.

Even when there is no obvious lymph node involvement in the armpit on exam or imaging, your surgeon will probably have performed a biopsy on at least one of these nodes during your surgery. (Older women with hormone receptor–positive breast cancers don't always need such a biopsy if the doctor already knows that the primary treatment will be with hormone therapies.) The surgeon will have injected a radioactive substance, or blue dye, or both, near the tumor and in the lymph nodes closest to the tumor (sentinel lymph nodes) so that they become visible. The surgeon removes these lymph nodes (also called a sentinel lymph node biopsy), and the pathologist checks for the presence of cancer cells. Your pathology report will include the number of nodes affected and whether they contain cancer cells. This information helps the doctor determine your stage.

Tumor Genomic Information

This sounds similar to genetic testing, but it is different. Genetic testing usually refers to the genes that you inherited from your mom and dad, also known as your germline DNA. This information is obtained from samples of your saliva or blood to test for the presence of certain genes that may predispose you to certain cancers. Tumor genomic testing, on the other hand, looks at the genes of the cancer tumors themselves and measures the activity of the genes in the tumor tissue.

The most widely used genomic test in early-stage breast cancer is called the Oncotype DX test. It provides information about how likely the cancer is to recur after treatment and whether you might need chemotherapy to give you a better chance at a cure. This test is appropriate for those with early-stage, estrogen receptor–positive, HER2-negative cancers.

This test will give you a number called a Recurrence Score. Your doctor will tell you whether she feels this number points to a low risk or a high risk of breast cancer recurrence. Those with a low-risk score won't need chemotherapy to prevent recurrence and will just be treated with hormone therapy. High-risk cancers would benefit from chemotherapy, and later hormonal therapy, to help prevent recurrence. There is some room for interpretation, and age along with your Recurrence Score may play a role in whether your doctor thinks you might benefit from the chemotherapy prior to hormone therapy.

Other Tests

If you have a larger tumor or one involving the lymph nodes of the armpit, it has a higher chance of spreading beyond the breast and lymph nodes. Your doctor may order additional lab or imaging studies to see if there may be cancer in other parts of your body. This may include checking blood work, CT scans, a bone scan, or possibly other imaging studies.

When your oncologist suspects there might be tumors in places other than your breast or armpit—for example, in the liver, bone, or lungs—they may recommend getting a biopsy of this area. This biopsy will tell us if this is breast cancer that has spread somewhere outside the breast and lymph nodes. It can also tell us the type, grade, and receptor status of that other tumor.

You may also have symptoms that seem unrelated to breast cancer, and your doctor might order a scan to check things out. For example, if a person has been experiencing persistent abdominal pain, a CT scan may show a spot that looks like cancer somewhere in the body, such as the liver, in addition to a breast mass. A biopsy of the suspicious spot may show that breast cancer has spread beyond the region of the breast to other parts of the body.

Recurring Breast Cancer

Occasionally, people who were successfully treated for breast cancer in months or years past may find that they have a new lump in their breast or armpit and are worried that their cancer has returned. In this case, the oncologist would perform an exam and order additional breast imaging if need be. Other persons with a history of an early-stage breast cancer may have persistent pain in their abdomen, or in a particular bone, or perhaps shortness of breath. In this situation, I would ask the patient to come to the clinic to talk about her symptoms. I would do an examination and discuss whether we should check body scans to see if there are signs that the cancer has returned. If scans show possible new tumors in other parts of her body, I would order a biopsy of these tumors to see if these are breast cancer cells. If this biopsy shows that the cancer has returned, we would discuss what treatment options might help.

I met Iris when she was 68 years old, after she had been successfully treated twice for breast cancer. She was first diagnosed at age 61 with an early-stage, ER-positive, HER2-negative cancer. After surgery, radiation, and hormone therapy, she was cancer free until age 64 when it came back in her lymph nodes. She had more surgery, radiation, and hormone therapy along with chemotherapy and was declared cancer free for a second time. After three years, she experienced terrible neck pain. When we checked scans of her neck and spine, we found spots that looked like bone metastases. A biopsy confirmed that it was breast cancer that had traveled to her bones. She started on treatment and is doing well years later.

What's My Stage?

My patients are eager to know the stage of their cancer as soon as possible. This is the question being posed by their loved ones and friends, which can be anxiety-provoking, and patients often ask me to help them understand what "stage" is in the first place. In general, the stage of your cancer tells us how far the cancer has advanced. Knowing the stage helps us predict whether the cancer is likely curable and how likely it is to recur.

At the time of diagnosis, many people know that there are four stages of breast cancer, just as there are for every other type of solid tumor. And like other tumors, breast cancer relies what we call the TNM staging system. It takes into account the size of the tumor (T), the number of lymph nodes (N) that contain cancer, and the presence or absence of metastases (M), which are other tumors outside the breast. What's different about breast cancer is that we have a few more pieces of information to include in staging. The grade of the tumor cells affects staging, and so does the receptor status.

Your oncologist will need to have a lot of information ready in order to determine your stage. The process of staging can be so complex that I have an app on my phone that allows me to plug in all of the diagnostic variables to determine the stage of a particular cancer. Sometimes your oncologist may know your stage during your initial consultation, and other times you may need to undergo more testing.

Stages 1, 2, and 3 (technically, this is written I, II, and III) are all potentially curable stages of breast cancer. We often say that a patient has an early-stage breast cancer if she has a smaller tumor (smaller than 5 centimeters) confined to the breast and with no or minimal lymph node involvement. A tumor is considered "locally advanced" if it is very large (larger than 5 centimeters), involves the skin of the breast or the muscles beneath the breast, or involves lots of lymph nodes in the armpit or above or below the collar bone. Inflammatory breast cancers are also considered locally advanced and describe a cancer that grows fast along the skin of the breast, making the breast red and swollen.

Stage 4 (IV) breast cancer, also known as metastatic breast cancer, is when the original tumor has moved to other sites in the body (called metastases). While breast cancer can metastasize to many different places, it most commonly spreads to the bone, lungs, liver, and brain. Most often metastatic breast cancer is not treated with surgery because surgery will not treat the tumors in other parts of the body. Metastatic breast cancer is most often treated with oral or intravenous treatments that can go throughout the body. The type of therapy will depend on many things, including the type of receptors the tumor has (estrogen, progesterone, and/or HER2). We will describe this in more detail later.

Currently, we do not have treatments that can rid the body of metastatic breast cancer; therefore, it is not generally thought to be curable. It is important to remember that with effective breast cancer therapies, many women may live well with the diagnosis of metastatic disease for several years.

The Goal of Treatment

One of the most important questions to ask your oncologist is "What is the goal of my treatment?" But we can talk about this only when we know the pathology and the staging. I've had patients blurt out in the first several seconds that they are never going to do chemotherapy, before they even know the diagnosis, stage, and treatment options. Or I've had patients say that they will do everything to fight the cancer and try to beat it. People and the media often talk about fighting cancer, but oncologists don't think in these terms. We think in terms of the goals of treatment, and there are just three:

1. *Cure the cancer.* This means using the standard treatments of surgery, radiation, and/or treatments that go throughout your body—such as hormonal therapy or chemotherapy—to kill or remove the cancer cells from your body.

2. *Prolong your life*. If your type of cancer can't be cured, your doctor will recommend treatments in the hope of giving you as much time as possible. Even when cancer can't be cured, it can often be controlled, meaning the growth of tumors can be slowed down, so that you will live longer.

3. *Make you feel better*. Even when your doctor knows that treatments won't cure you or prolong your life, he or she may recommend treatments that will make you much more comfortable.

Nothing should be prescribed for you unless it fits at least one of these stated goals. Again: to try to cure the cancer, to prolong your life, and/or to make you feel better. What does your doctor think is possible for you? What are your goals and values? Which of the possible treatments feel right for you? How much treatment do you want? How intensive can those treatments be while allowing you to maintain your quality of life? By knowing the goal of treatment, you can better choose treatment options that are right for you.

Your Goals and Values

Sometimes the goal of treatment changes when people find out what it will take to have a chance at a cure. I recently treated two very similar women with triple-negative breast cancers. Both Margaret and Flo were in their early seventies and in excellent health. I told each of them that with surgery and radiation, there was a 70% chance that their cancers would be cured. If we added chemotherapy, the likelihood of a cure would improve by about 10%. Margaret was very clear that she wanted chemotherapy, because she hoped to have the chance to see her granddaughter complete nursing school in the next few years. Flo decided against chemotherapy. She did not think that the burdens and side effects of chemotherapy were worth an additional 10% chance of being cured. She also had a busy year ahead that included an important family wedding and a dream trip abroad. She knew that months of chemotherapy might not allow her to enjoy these important events with her family. This is what I mean by making treatment decisions that are right for you and your life goals. There aren't any right answers, only right answers for you.

If the doctor tells you that your cancer isn't curable, you still have choices about what treatments to use to control the cancer. Treatments such as chemotherapy and radiation are disruptive, and you will need to think about what you want to endure to prolong your life. Some people view living as long as they possibly can as the ultimate goal, while others prefer to emphasize living as well as they can. One of my patients with metastatic hormone receptor–positive breast cancer was clear from our first visit that she wanted to minimize her time at the hospital and did not want to be treated with chemotherapy. We were able to use hormonal therapies for years to keep her breast cancer stable, but when the cancer eventually progressed she elected to enroll in hospice, even though chemotherapy may have prolonged her life by several months or even a year. She felt that the extra time chemotherapy may have bought her was not worth the side effects and the additional visits to the hospital. Ultimately, she lived well for several months at home, enjoying time with her family and touching base with me by phone to give me updates.

Knowing the goal of treatment as well as your values empowers you throughout therapy. It gives you the ability to choose treatments that help you achieve your goals and to decline treatments that won't. Early on, you may want to pursue every treatment to have a chance at curing a cancer or to prolong your life. Over time, that goal may change, and that's okay too.

The Treatment Plan

Once your doctor tells you what your type of cancer is and the stage, he or she may talk about a plan for treatment. Just as there are only three goals of cancer treatment (cure, live longer, feel better), there are three broad options to treat a cancer:

1. *Standard therapy*, using recognized, proven therapies studied by oncologists, designed to eradicate the cancer or keep it in check for as long as possible.

2. *Experimental therapy*, which involves clinical trials. Some clinical trials may involve newer, less-proven therapies, while other clinical trials are evaluating standard regimens.

3. *Supportive care alone*, which will keep you comfortable and active for as long as possible or simply monitor for the possible recurrence of cancer.

It's my job as an oncologist to work with you to learn about your goals and values so that we can think through these different treatment plans together, to see what matches best to what matters most to you. I recently treated a young woman with an early-stage hormone receptor–positive, HER2-negative breast cancer with chemotherapy, and we discussed adding an experimental therapy to her standard hormonal therapy. She said that she knew the extra visits, labs, and radiology testing would bring on an incredible amount of anxiety for her, and she decided that the clinical trial was not the right choice for her. I have also been following another young woman in her fifties with a hormone receptor–positive, HER2-negative metastatic breast cancer whose cancer had progressed despite multiple standard hormonal therapies and chemotherapies, as well as experimental therapies over the preceding years. She was not eligible for any additional experimental therapies, and we discussed the low but possible benefit from one more standard chemotherapy (5%) or transitioning to supportive care alone. She and her husband were clear in their goal of trying any therapy that might have even a remote chance of prolonging her life. She decided to try additional therapy and planned to transition to supportive care when this treatment stopped working.

Oncologic Emergencies

Even soon after a cancer diagnosis, emergencies can occur. At any time in your treatment, if you experience any of the symptoms in table 2.1, call your doctor or the clinic immediately, regardless of the time. In these instances, you want a call back from a clinician within 10 to 15 minutes. If you don't hear back from a clinician and are feeling unwell, you should go to the emergency room.

Choosing a New Oncologist

Sometimes patients and families wonder about switching oncologists or getting a second opinion. You may have met with an oncologist who didn't seem to be a good match for you. Sometimes you really like and trust your oncologist but would feel more comfortable having another opinion. This may feel awkward, but it happens a lot. Your oncologist wants you to feel comfortable with your care. You have the right to feel that you have explored all available options. Vicki, Dave, and I encourage our patients to seek out whatever information they need, and I tell them that whether they transition to another oncologist or come back to see me, I just want them to feel comfortable with their care.

When you look for another oncologist or opinion, you will want to find someone who specializes in breast cancer or who has treated a lot of people with breast cancer. Because breast cancer is so common, this is not usually difficult to do. Some people want a doctor who is prominent in the field, but for others, that may not be as important as finding someone who is a good communicator. You want to work with a doctor who invites questions and answers them, someone who sees you as a person, someone you can call at any time, someone you trust. You also want to work with someone who is part of a well-staffed team so there are nurse practitioners or physician assistants, nurses, social workers, and other team members who can talk to you any time and see you right away when you need advice and help. Ultimately, you want to find an oncologist and a team who can support you—who will get to know you and what matters most to you. You want a team who will collaborate on treatments that match your goals and values, pay attention to your quality of life, and assist you in navigating cancer care.

Table 2.1. Oncological emergencies

Sign or symptom	What it might indicate
Fever ≥100.4 degrees Fahrenheit (38 degrees Celsius) in the setting of chemotherapy	Possible low white blood cell count (febrile neutropenia) and the need for antibiotics
Fever ≥100.4 degrees Fahrenheit (38 degrees Celsius) and shaking chills	Possible bacteria in the bloodstream
New confusion	Possible brain metastasis or serious side effects from medications
Back pain with neurologic symptoms (leg weakness or rubberiness; difficulty holding bladder or bowels)	Possible spinal cord compression
Swelling of the neck and face with distended veins	Main veins in the neck may be blocked (superior vena cava syndrome)
Acute chest pain, particularly when taking in a deep breath, with or without shortness of breath	Possible blood clot in the lungs (pulmonary embolus)

CHAPTER THREE

Local Therapies in Breast Cancer

When Vicki, Dave, or I sit down with a new patient for the first time, we often have to explain that there may be three separate types of oncologists involved in their care. I'm a medical oncologist, which means that I prescribe chemotherapy and hormonal therapies that treat the cancer throughout the whole body. I also help with symptoms and side effects of both the cancer and its treatment. If you've been diagnosed with an early-stage breast cancer, you might also need to see a surgical oncologist, who specializes in removing breast cancer tumors. Many people also need a radiation oncologist, who specializes in using radiation to treat cancer cells that might remain in the breast and lymph nodes after surgery. Some women with advanced breast cancer may also see a radiation oncologist to treat metastases that are causing pain or symptoms. Each of these doctors will treat you individually, and they will also be communicating with each other to ensure that they are creating a plan to best care for you. Doctors refer to surgery and radiation as local therapies because they work to remove cancer cells at a specific site.

In this chapter, I'll talk about the types of surgery and radiation your doctor may be recommending and what you can expect from each.

Types of Breast Surgery

If you have been diagnosed with a stage 1, 2, or 3 breast cancer, your surgeon will talk to you about the options for surgery. Depending on the diagnosis or stage of the cancer, he or she may recommend removing the tumor alone or the entire breast. In some cases, your medical team will recommend chemotherapy, anti-HER2 treatments, or hormonal therapy before surgery. When your oncologist recommends these treatments prior to surgery, he or she may be hoping to shrink the tumor and increase the chances that the tumor can be removed with clean margins. Perhaps shrinking a tumor will allow for a lumpectomy rather than a mastectomy. In some cases, these treatments give important information about how responsive the tumor is to therapy, so your doctor knows whether more treatments are needed after surgery.

Lumpectomy

This type of surgery is also sometimes called breast-conserving surgery. With a lumpectomy, the surgeon removes the tumor and a rim of normal tissue around the tumor. A pathologist will examine the cells of the normal tissue to see if it is free from cancer. If it contains no cancerous cells, you will be told that you have clear or negative margins, which is great news. If the margins are not clear, your team will likely discuss an additional surgery to remove a little more breast tissue, called a re-excision. Sometimes, the surgeon may recommend a mastectomy.

The benefit of a lumpectomy is that it's a less invasive procedure with a shorter recovery time. You will be able to keep your breast and in most cases the cosmetic results are good or even excellent, with the treated breast looking similar to the untreated breast. The downside is that, in most cases, you will have to have some radiation treatment afterward. There is data to support leaving out radiation in women over the age of 65–70 who have small tumors that are hormone receptor–positive. If you are in this age group and have no lymph node involvement, your doctor may omit radiation therapy as long as you take the recommended hormonal therapy. Another downside of lumpectomy is that there are slightly higher rates of the breast tumor recurring within that same breast. If this happens, your medical team will probably recommend a mastectomy. The good news is, if you have a lumpectomy followed by radiation, your survival rate is the same as someone who had a mastectomy.

Lumpectomy is an option for most who have early-stage breast cancer. Though some who have this option do choose mastectomy instead. It is perfectly normal to struggle with this decision. During the course of a week, it is not uncommon for me to meet two women with an early-stage breast cancer who view this decision from very different perspectives. For example, Emily is a 50-year-old woman who was diagnosed with a stage 1 hormone receptor–positive, HER2-negative breast cancer who knew immediately she wanted to proceed with bilateral mastectomies. She said that she tended to be a worrier, and even though she understood that more surgery would not increase her survival, she would sleep better at night with a mastectomy. At around the same time, I met Ann who had a similar tumor but opted for lumpectomy because she really wanted to preserve her own breast and did not want to consider reconstruction options.

If you are unsure of which surgery is right for you, ask yourself some questions: Do I hope to keep my breast? Am I hoping that my breasts will match in size? How anxious am I about the possibility of a recurrence? Am I willing to be treated with radiation after a lumpectomy? Ask your surgeon questions about the advantages and disadvantages of each surgery and let her know what things are most important to you as you make your decision.

Mastectomy

A mastectomy is removal of the entire breast. It may be recommended due to the size or location of your tumor or due to the size of the tumor relative to the size of your breast. For example, if your breast is small but the tumor is large, there may be no cosmetic reason to conserve the remaining tissue with a lumpectomy. If you have separate tumors in different quadrants of the breast, a mastectomy is often recommended. Some women may be offered a lumpectomy but may prefer to undergo a mastectomy.

Genetic mutations and medical conditions may weigh into the decision for a mastectomy as well. Women with genetic mutations placing them at risk for another breast cancer (such as BRCA1 or BRCA2) may elect to have a mastectomy. There are also some medical conditions like Li-Fraumeni syndrome and connective tissue diseases like lupus where radiation may not be advised. In these individuals, the surgeon may recommend a mastectomy. And there are three different types:

1. *Simple mastectomy.* This type of surgery is usually recommended for women who don't have cancer cells or tumors in the lymph nodes of the armpit. The surgeon removes the entire breast and will likely do a biopsy of the lymph node closest to the tumor (sentinel lymph node) at the same time.

2. *Modified radical mastectomy.* If a biopsy has confirmed that some lymph nodes contain cancer, you might have this surgery. It removes the entire breast as well as some lymph nodes in the armpit.

3. *Contralateral prophylactic mastectomy.* This is also called a preventative mastectomy. Some women decide to remove the opposite breast that does not have cancer. For patients who have a genetic predisposition to breast cancer, because of a BRCA1 or BRCA2 mutation, a

prophylactic mastectomy can reduce the risk of getting a breast cancer in the breast that does not yet have cancer. For those women who don't have such a mutation or hereditary risk factors for breast cancer, a preventative mastectomy has little or no effect on survival. Still, some women elect for this procedure because they worry about developing another breast cancer. Or they hope to undergo reconstructive surgery in both breasts to allow for symmetry.

Breast Reconstruction

Breast reconstruction is surgery to restore the shape of your breast after a mastectomy. Your surgeon will talk to you about whether you would like to undergo breast reconstruction and what types of reconstruction options are available to you. Some women don't wish to have breast reconstruction. They may opt instead for a breast prosthesis that sits inside the bra to help provide the contour of a breast beneath their clothing. Others who don't pursue breast reconstruction may decide to go without a breast prosthesis, sometimes called "going flat" or "living flat."

Your surgeon may offer the choice of reconstruction done at the time of the mastectomy, or at a later date. For patients who choose an immediate reconstruction, it may be possible to have a skin-sparing mastectomy, in which the surgeon removes the nipple and areola, but leaves the skin over the breast intact. In some cases, the surgeon may also be able to leave the nipple, areola, or both. However, if the tumor involves the skin, nipple, or areola, the surgeon will need to remove these tissues.

Choosing breast reconstruction is a very personal decision, and it is helpful to hear from both the breast surgeon and plastic surgeon about the different options. Ask what the breast might look like after surgery and about the recovery time. You will want to know if you will have radiation treatments and how those might affect the timing of the surgery and the look of the reconstructed breast. And you will want to know about possible complications in the short and long term.

There are a number of techniques available to reconstruct your breast:

1. *Breast implant.* These are devices inserted under the skin to recreate the breast shape. All implants have a shell surface that is made of silicone and then filled with either saline or silicone. Saline implants are filled with sterile salt water. They tend to feel firmer but may show more wrinkling under the skin when compared to silicone implants.

Silicone gel implants tend to feel softer than saline implants, and some people feel that silicone implants have a more natural look and feel. Both have a small risk of rupturing, requiring surgery to place another implant.

Sometimes the implant is put in at the same time as the mastectomy. Other times there is a two-step process involving an expander to stretch the skin and muscle in the chest after which the surgeon adds small amounts of fluid into the expander over time. Eventually the expander is removed and a breast implant is inserted.

2. *Flap procedures*. The surgeon may be able to use your own body tissue to reconstruct the breast. Because these procedures use your own tissue, the reconstructed breasts feel more natural. However, flap surgeries are longer and more involved than implant surgeries. In a TRAM flap procedure, the surgeon removes part of the transverse rectus abdominis muscle (TRAM) as well as some abdominal fat and skin tissue to form a new breast. Because the procedure cuts into muscles that you would normally use for sit-ups, you may lose some abdominal strength after the surgery. The DIEP flap procedure instead uses tissue from the lower abdomen (deep inferior epigastric perforator, or DIEP), which means that your abdominal muscles will be intact afterward. Latissimus dorsi flaps use tissue from the upper back.

Whether and what type of flap procedure may be possible depends on many factors, such as how much extra body fat you have and where it is located, as well as your overall health. Some centers have more expertise in flap surgeries and may offer this more frequently to their patients. So, it's best to have a detailed discussion with a breast and plastic surgeon about your options. If your center does not do many flap surgeries and you are interested in finding out whether this might be an option for you, you might consider seeking out another opinion.

3. *Nipple reconstruction*. If the surgeon removed the nipple and areola with the breast, it may be possible to reconstruct them, but this surgery usually takes place a few months after reconstruction. To reconstruct a nipple, the surgeon may be able to rearrange the tissue that is already there or may transfer fat from another part of your body to use for the reconstruction. Nipple and areola tattooing can help the reconstructed breast look more like the original breast.

Side Effects of Surgery

How you recover from surgery will depend on the type of surgery you have, and recovery periods can vary even among patients who have had the same surgery. Here are some of the side effects to be aware of.

Pain

In the days and short weeks after surgery, there may be pain and discomfort from having just had a surgical procedure. For many people, over-the-counter medications like acetaminophen and ibuprofen may be adequate to control this pain. Others may find that the addition of a short-course of stronger pain medication, such as opioids, may help them in the recovery process. A medication called gabapentin targets symptoms from the nerve damage that occurs during surgery and may help in the short term with any sharp, shooting nerve pain that you may experience afterward.

If you experience a lot more pain than you expect, or if you notice redness, warmth, or swelling in the area where you had surgery, you should call your surgeon. Sometimes women may have a buildup of fluid in the surgical area—called a seroma—that might need to be drained. Other times there may be an infection developing, and it is important that your surgical team evaluates you.

Some women experience pain or discomfort at the surgical site for months or even years after surgery. This can be very normal because surgery involves cutting across your tissues and nerves. Sometimes, even after healing, a person may experience intermittent discomfort, especially if pressure is applied to the area. Sometimes even years after surgery a strong bear hug can hurt. Of course, you will be undergoing regular visits with your doctor who will be examining you to check if anything else might be causing your pain.

Lymphedema

One or two lymph nodes may be removed from your armpit to look for cancer, and several more may be removed if there is a concern that the lymph nodes harbor more extensive amounts of cancer. Removing lymph nodes can disrupt the normal lymph drainage in your arm, and this can lead to swelling in the arm. This does not always happen, and it is more likely to happen when more lymph nodes are removed. Having radiation after surgery also increases the risk of lymphedema. There is a machine called a perometer that measures the circumference of your arm, and your doctor may follow these measurements over time to assess whether there is a difference between your two arms or to assess the amount of lymphedema present.

Some doctors advise that patients avoid blood draws and blood pressure cuffs in this area. There is reassuring data, however, that blood draws and cuffs may not increase the risk of lymphedema. So, if you feel better avoiding these things, that is okay. However, you can be reassured that they do not likely cause much harm.

Mobility Issues

Sometimes the ability to fully extend your arm in all directions might be limited by breast surgery or the radiation after surgery. This is more common when you've had more extensive surgery and radiation. If this happens, your surgeon will likely give you instructions for some simple exercises that will help increase your range of motion. Sometimes, it is helpful to work with a physical therapist to decrease some of the tightness in the breast and armpit area and to increase your mobility. For example, Nadine was being treated for stage 3 triple-negative breast cancer. She had a mastectomy that required the removal of 10 lymph nodes in her armpit. After surgery, she experienced some decreased mobility of her right arm, making it harder for her to garden. We referred her for physical therapy, which helped increase her mobility significantly and allowed her to feel more comfortable in her garden. Later that year, after chemotherapy and radiation, Nadine started to experience some swelling in her right arm from lymphedema, so she went back to physical therapy. The physical therapist fit her for a lymphedema compression sleeve, which she uses at night, and she now has very minimal swelling in the arm.

Coping with a New Body

Women have different reactions to breast surgery. Some women feel pleased with the cosmetic results of their breast surgery and do not feel differently about their bodies or their sexuality. But this isn't true for everyone. For many women it takes time to get used to the way they look after surgery and radiation. The changes might be dramatic, or they might not be noticeable to others but very noticeable to you. For many the surgery is a reminder of cancer treatment and all that may have changed as a result of the cancer diagnosis and treatment. We'll talk more about coping with your new body in chapter 7.

Surgery for Metastatic Breast Cancer

It's uncommon for people with metastatic breast cancer to be treated with surgery because it doesn't treat the disease that has spread beyond the original tumor. The best way to get treatment to the other tumor sites is through systemic treatments (treatments that reach the entire body), such as chemotherapy, hormonal therapy, or targeted therapies. Still, your doctor may consider surgery if a tumor is causing significant symptoms that may be hard to control with other therapies. For example, I cared for a 65-year-old woman named Annette with a hormone receptor–positive, HER2-negative metastatic breast cancer. She was first diagnosed because of shortness of breath. During her examination and testing, her doctor found that she had anemia from a large bleeding breast tumor that had likely been present for several years. Annette had a mastectomy to control the bleeding, and she underwent radiation afterward. Over the years, she had some slow progression of the tumor in her chest wall, but the surgery and radiation helped her symptoms and provided her with years of disease control. I also care for another patient named Nadia, a 76-year-old woman who was treated for a hormone receptor–positive, HER2-negative breast cancer 15 years prior who called me because she could not lift up her right foot. We checked an MRI of her spine and found a bulky, large tumor in her sacral region. The orthopedic surgery team removed some of the tumor pressing on her nerves with the goal of helping restore and preserve her function. In both of these cases, the surgery helped control symptoms in order to restore quality of life.

What Is Radiation Therapy?

Radiation therapy uses x-rays (also called photons) to kill cancer cells. Because cancer cells grow quickly, they are more prone to the damage from radiation therapy than are normal cells. Radiation kills cancer cells by damaging their DNA. If the cells have enough radiation damage, they will die when they try to divide.

There are two types of conventional radiation therapy: external and internal. The most common form of radiation therapy for breast cancer is external beam radiation. A machine called a linear accelerator produces a beam, or a series of beams, of x-rays that target the area of cancer in your body. For internal radiation therapy—also called brachytherapy—a radiation oncologist places a temporary device that holds radioactive seeds inside the breast at the location of the tumor.

Conventional radiation uses x-rays that enter and exit the body. A radiation oncologist can "paint" the radiation around the tumor to try and limit the normal tissues receiving radiation. Proton beam therapy, on the other hand, delivers a narrow concentration of radiation to the tumor. It is not more effective at killing the cancer, but it may be better at limiting the side effects of radiation to other parts of the body. Studies are underway comparing x-rays to protons. In general, proton beam therapy is not considered standard care and is not usually offered unless a patient is enrolled in a clinical trial.

There are different approaches to radiation. The first is called whole breast irradiation, in which the entire breast is treated. This course of radiation is usually delivered daily for four weeks. A second type of radiation is called regional nodal irradiation, in which the entire breast or chest wall is treated along with the lymph nodes that sit around the breast. This course of radiation is usually delivered for five to six weeks.

The third type is called accelerated partial breast irradiation (APBI), and it uses slightly higher doses of radiation focused on a smaller region of the breast where the tumor was removed. Because of the smaller volume of tissue, this course of radiation is often delivered over a shorter period of time, typically one to two weeks, with a slightly higher dose delivered at each treatment. This option is typically reserved for patients with early-stage and low-risk breast cancer.

Do I Need Radiation?

Radiation can be used in early-stage breast cancer to reduce the risk of breast cancer recurring after surgery, and it is usually recommended after a lumpectomy. Your medical team may recommend radiation therapy even after a mastectomy. This is particularly true when tumors are larger or when they have invaded some lymph nodes.

Radiation is used to treat the microscopic cancer cells that may remain around the site after the tumor has been removed. Even if a surgeon has removed all of the tumor tissue, patients can still be at risk of another tumor developing from microscopic cells that were left behind. Some cancers are like jellyfish in that they grow tentacles outward from the central tumor and these can't be seen on scans. Your doctor may want to use radiation to have a better chance of killing those cells.

Your team may also recommend radiation if you have metastatic breast cancer because it can reduce the symptoms and growth from metastatic cancer. In fact, it can be a helpful way to reduce or eliminate pain from metastatic sites, including bone metastases. If a breast mass is growing and breaking through the skin, causing ulceration and bleeding, your doctors may recommend radiation to help control your symptoms. It can also stop cancers from bleeding or growing into vital structures like the spinal cord or liver. If the cancer has spread to the brain, radiation therapy can treat the tumor site or the whole brain.

The Planning Session

Everyone who gets radiation therapy undergoes a planning session, often called a simulation, or "sim." This planning session typically takes less than an hour to complete. The radiation oncologist and radiation therapist will position your body in a way that is both comfortable and reproducible for you and that permits the safest delivery of radiation to the area of the body they wish to treat, while also avoiding the parts of your body that should not receive radiation. They will take a CT scan of your body in this position and the pictures from the scan are then used to plan out exactly where the radiation will enter and exit your body. By using multiple beams of radiation, the radiation oncologist can often concentrate the highest dose around the cancer and limit the amount normal tissues receive.

When they have figured out the appropriate position for your body, they will often place a few small tattoos on the skin as a reference point. This ensures that the radiation therapist can position you correctly for each session of radiation, which is critical to delivering therapy to the proper location. The tattoo is usually a small blue dot the size of a pen mark. If you have tumors in the brain, you might need to be fitted with a radiation mask instead of getting tattoos. The mask will be used with each radiation treatment to make sure that the beam is in exactly the right position. The radiation oncology team will discuss all of this with you and take you through it step by step. It can sound daunting, but once you learn the ropes and get to know your team, it will all feel easier.

How Much Radiation Will I Need?

You may be scheduled to receive either a long course or a short course of radiation. In a long course, smaller amounts of radiation are delivered every day over an extended time, perhaps four to six weeks. In short-course radiation therapy, larger doses of radiation are delivered every day over an abbreviated period, such as one week.

The dose of radiation that any patient receives is measured in Gray, named after Henry Louis Gray, one of the pioneers in x-ray technology. A Gray is often abbreviated Gy. Each Gy is equivalent to one joule of energy absorbed per kilogram of tissue. The total amount of Gy used after breast surgery to kill breast cancer cells varies depending on the technique but may be in the range of 40 to 50 Gy. By comparison, a CT scan has 16 milligray, or .016 Gy. The amount of radiation delivered with each daily dose is called a fraction, and this is also measured in Gy.

You will typically need to arrive for radiation at the same time each day, and you will usually have the same radiation therapists to position you on the table and direct the radiation based on the location the radiation oncologist is trying to treat. The radiation itself lasts only a few minutes, but the entire visit to the radiation oncology department will generally take 30 to 45 minutes. Like everything else, you will get used to the routine, and the staff will be able to get you in and out pretty quickly. I have had many patients tell me that they become friendly with the other patients getting radiation at the same time because you may see each other every day for up to several weeks. You become radiation buddies. When you complete a course of radiation, many hospitals have a bell in the waiting room that you can ring if you want. It becomes a celebratory moment to mark completion of the course.

Side Effects of Radiation

As with many cancer therapies, it is hard to know how each individual might tolerate radiation. Some people go through radiation feeling relatively well, while others may experience more side effects. Some women may have recently gone through surgery and chemotherapy and are still dealing with some of the side effects from these treatments as they enter into radiation therapy.

These are the potential short- and long-term side effects to radiation to take note of:

Fatigue. This is one of the more common immediate side effects of radiation. You may get tired about two weeks after the radiation starts, and this may last for a few weeks after it ends. Compared to fatigue experienced after chemotherapy, this fatigue is usually mild. This will usually subside over the course of about a month, but I encourage people to think about how they will manage this fatigue so they are prepared. Some people may find naps helpful, and while many people work full-time during radiation, it may be helpful to have some flexibility in your schedule, if possible.

Inflammation. Although the treatment itself is painless, radiation does cause some short-term swelling in soft tissues. This swelling can cause discomfort, but it is generally temporary. If your breast or armpit area is being radiated, you may develop what looks like a sunburn in this area, called radiation dermatitis. Sometimes, the skin peels off and becomes more raw, like a severe sunburn. The radiation team will talk to you about using skin moisturizers from the start and may modify these recommendations if your skin becomes more inflamed.

Scarring. The normal tissues in the path of radiation beams can sustain long-term damage. For women who receive radiation to the underarm for breast cancer, this scarring can cause the affected arm to swell and cause lymphedema. If radiation has hit the digestive tract, you can get scarring that causes obstructions there. Occasionally, vital organs can be scarred, including the heart and kidneys, and this can lead to long-term damage. Typically, if this happens, it takes place slowly, months or years after radiation is complete. This isn't usually a concern among breast cancer patients unless metastases in other parts of the body are being treated. Radiation oncologists do everything they can to avoid vital organs, but sometimes the location of the tumor doesn't allow for this.

Bone marrow suppression. Radiation can damage the stem cells in your bone marrow, which can impair the production of blood cells in your body. If you are receiving radiation to the breast, bone marrow suppression is unlikely, but if you are receiving radiation to your bones, it may be more of a concern. Usually your body can bounce back after radiation has stopped and your bone marrow has had some time to recover.

Pneumonitis. Even though radiation to the breast and armpit is focused to those areas, sometimes a small amount of radiation will reach a small portion of the lungs. In rare cases, this can cause pneumonitis, or inflammation of the lung. And if it does occur, it is typically in the months following radiation. This can sometimes be serious, and if you experience a cough or shortness of breath, you should call your oncologist. Sometimes we need to treat pneumonitis with a few weeks of steroids.

Cancer. The risk of developing a new radiation -induced cancer in the area that was radiated is approximately 0.5% over the course of the next 20 years. Still, this is a serious consideration that must be weighed against the beneficial effects of radiation for treating cancer.

Again, it is difficult to predict which side effects you may experience with radiation therapy. How you respond to therapy depends on which part of the body is being treated, as well as the length and strength of radiation. Your overall health plays a role here as does the number of treatments you've been through. And sometimes it's just chance.

My patient Rochelle had a lumpectomy followed by chemotherapy. Despite having been a really healthy, active woman prior to the cancer diagnosis, she needed a lot of support in chemotherapy to combat the side effects of fatigue, joint pains, and some tingling in her hands and feet. Afterward she was scheduled for a short course of radiation and she worried aloud about the possibility of more fatigue. She told me she was tired of feeling wiped out all the time. We were both relieved when she sailed through the radiation with good energy and was able to go back to work. I suspect that her body simply tolerated the radiation better than the chemotherapy. Many women like Rochelle tolerate radiation really well and are often able to maintain most of their normal routine, including working, during radiation treatments.

Some patients are surprised to feel poorly during radiation therapy because the treatment is so targeted to the breast. Arlene is an otherwise healthy 55-year-old woman with stage 1 breast cancer who had a lumpectomy followed by radiation. She experienced so much fatigue from radiation therapy that she requested time off from work. As an attorney who loves to work long days and take long power walks with her dogs, she was not prepared to feel so tired. Fortunately, within a month of completing radiation , she was back to her routine and felt that most of her energy had returned.

Why Am I Not Getting Surgery or Radiation?

Not every patient diagnosed with breast cancer is a good candidate for local therapies. If you have been diagnosed with metastatic cancer or recurring cancer, your doctor might not recommend surgery or radiation. This can be confusing. I've had patients ask me why they aren't scheduled for surgery to remove a breast tumor. When there are tumors in areas beyond the breast and armpit, surgery and radiation are not able to treat the cancer in the other areas of the body and so are not the most effective treatments overall. Your doctor will instead be focusing on systemic treatments such as chemotherapy and hormonal treatments. These can treat the cancer throughout your body. We will review those therapies in the next chapter.

CHAPTER FOUR

How to Prepare for Systemic Treatment

Starting treatment can be unnerving because you don't know what to expect and because this is when you become a patient being treated for cancer. You may have been diagnosed with an early-stage breast cancer and recently had surgery. Or you may have been told that chemotherapy, rather than surgery, is the first step to treating your cancer. Everything may feel surreal, and you may just be starting to wrap your mind around the idea of having cancer in the first place. This time is also one of the toughest because you don't know how your body is going to respond to treatment. You don't yet know how to trust this new body, but you will. You will become a competent, capable cancer patient. We wish you didn't have to, but you will.

In this chapter, I (Jenn) am going to talk you through everything you need to know to prepare for breast cancer treatments. I talked about the local therapies that may be used to treat breast cancer in chapter 3 and will focus now on what we call the systemic therapies to treat breast cancer. These are drugs that travel throughout the body to treat cancer cells. The types of treatment that you receive depend on a lot of factors, including the stage and subtype of tumor that you have.

Even though you won't likely need all of these treatments, an introduction to the general categories of treatment will give you an understanding of what you can expect from them. First, I'll explain the most common classes of breast cancer treatments and how they work, including a typical day in the infusion unit, which is the facility inside the hospital or clinic where chemotherapy is provided. I'll also tell you what you need to know about side effects, and how you can adjust your schedule for chemotherapy to better fit into your life.

What Are the Common Systemic Therapies?

Systemic breast cancer therapies can be subdivided into four major categories: hormonal therapy, chemotherapy, targeted therapy, and immunotherapy. Each of these categories carries different side effects that can be easy or difficult to tolerate, and each can be administered in several ways. They can be given intravenously (through a vein), orally (by mouth), subcutaneously (under the skin), or intramuscularly (in the muscle). It is important to note, too, that breast cancer therapies are constantly changing. New drugs may be approved, and sometimes a drug that may have been used to treat only metastatic cancer is now being used to treat early-stage cancer as well. I cover the general categories of systemic therapies here to give you an understanding of the treatments more broadly, and specific treatment examples can be found in tables 4.1 and 4.2.

Hormonal Therapy

These drugs kill breast cancer cells that are dependent on being fed from hormones in your body, specifically estrogen. Unlike chemotherapy, most hormonal therapies (sometimes called endocrine therapy) are oral treatments. These treatments include drugs such as tamoxifen and the aromatase inhibitors (anastrozole, letrozole, and exemestane). Fulvestrant and drugs to suppress the ovaries (such as leuprolide) are hormonal therapies that are injected into the muscle. The side effects are often quite manageable when compared with traditional chemotherapy, but these treatments can cause such problems as early menopause, hot flashes, joint and muscle aches, osteoporosis, changes in mood and libido, and other long-term complications caused by low estrogen.

While it is rare to have a life-threatening complication from hormonal therapy, these side effects can be very disruptive. Sometimes patients feel that their oncologists may not pay enough attention to their complaints about these deeply personal bodily changes. Other times, patients may feel embarrassed about talking to an oncologist about these symptoms. You can ask your oncologist to refer you to a member of the medical team who specializes in managing the symptoms of menopause, or you can talk to your own gynecologist about ways to cope with your changing hormones. In some cases, palliative care specialists can also be a good resource. In chapter 8, we talk more about the side effects of hormonal treatments and what you can do to minimize them.

Chemotherapy

This is the cancer therapy with which most people are familiar. These drugs kill cancer cells usually by damaging their DNA in some way. Most chemotherapy to treat breast cancer is given intravenously. Capecitabine is the one chemotherapy that is given orally. Chemotherapy can cause well-known side effects, including nausea, hair loss, low blood counts, and fatigue. The side effects of each regimen do vary, and your doctor will go into the specific side effects for each one prescribed to you. There are several different chemotherapy regimens that are used to increase cure rates in early-stage breast cancer (see table 4.1) and many chemotherapies that are used to treat metastatic cancer (see table 4.2). I'll describe much more about chemotherapy later in the chapter.

In patients with early-stage cancer, chemotherapy may be given before surgery (neoadjuvant chemotherapy) or after surgery (adjuvant chemotherapy). From the surgeon's perspective, neoadjuvant chemotherapy may be used to shrink a larger tumor to a size that allows for a more successful surgery. A surgeon may not be able to remove a large, locally advanced tumor, but if the tumor shrinks with chemotherapy, she may be able to perform surgery. Other tumors may be too large to remove with a lumpectomy, but after chemotherapy they may shrink to a size where lumpectomy and radiation may be an option. In women with HER2-positive or triple-negative breast cancers, the medical oncologist may prefer to start with neoadjuvant chemotherapy.

After neoadjuvant therapy, you will still need to undergo surgery. If the treatment has been so effective that the pathologist can't find any remaining cancer cells in the breast or lymph node tissue that is removed, this is called a pathologic complete response, or pCR. In those with HER2-positive or triple-negative breast cancers, this information is particularly helpful. If a pCR is achieved in these patients, this is a good prognostic sign, and many studies have shown an association between pCR and better outcomes, like decreased recurrence and improved overall survival. If there was not a pCR (because there is still some cancer found at the time of surgery), the oncologist may recommend additional chemotherapy treatments (for example, capecitabine for triple-negative breast cancer and ado-trastuzumab emtansine for HER2-positive breast cancer; see table 4.1).

Targeted Therapy

These medications target the specific aspects of cancer cells that cause them to grow out of control. These treatments are more precise in blocking the growth of cancer cells. This is different from chemotherapy, which disrupts all fast-growing cells throughout the body and therefore causes more side effects. Targeted therapies usually cause fewer side effects, but they are only effective for specific types of cancer cells. Your diagnosis and the genetic makeup of your cells will determine if these drugs are an option for you. Targeted therapies can be prescribed alone, or they may be used in combination with chemotherapy or hormonal therapy. The most common targeted therapies for each subtype of breast cancer are listed here.

Hormone receptor–positive breast cancer. If you have a metastatic breast cancer that is also hormone receptor–positive, there are targeted therapies that may make the hormonal therapy more effective with the goal of helping you to feel better and live longer. These drugs (palbociclib, ribociclib, and abemaciclib) are called CDK4/6 inhibitors because they block proteins in breast cancer cells that promote growth. While sometimes these drugs can be used by themselves, more often these oral drugs are used along with such hormonal therapies as aromatase inhibitors (letrozole or anastrozole) or fulvestrant. Abemaciclib may also be used to treat some early-stage, higher-risk hormone receptor–positive breast cancers.

Similar to CDK4/6 inhibitors, drugs that inhibit a protein pathway in breast cancer cells called mTOR (mammalian target of rapamycin) can also be used along with hormonal drugs to treat metastatic breast cancer.

Doctors found that breast cancer mutations in a gene called PI3K (also sometimes called PIK3CA) can be targeted with specific drugs. In patients with metastatic hormone receptor–positive breast cancer, your doctor may check for a PIK3CA mutation in the tumor sample or in your blood. About 40% of hormone receptor–positive breast cancers have this mutation, and these mutations contribute to tumor resistance to hormonal therapies. The drug alpelisib can be used along with the hormonal therapy fulvestrant, and it can increase the impact of hormonal therapy.

HER2-positive breast cancer. HER2 is an important protein pathway in breast cancer cells that acts like a fuel line to breast cancer cells. When this protein pathway is turned on in a breast cancer cell, the cell grows more rapidly and can spread more easily throughout the body. We can tell whether this pathway is turned on in a person's breast cancer by measuring how much of the protein is on the surface of the breast cancer cell. About 20% of breast cancers have this pathway turned on and it's important for patients to be treated with drugs that turn this pathway off. The drugs listed in table 4.1 have clear benefits to breast cancer patients and have been shown in multiple clinical trials to help women with localized breast cancer be cured more often and women with metastatic breast cancer to live much longer and feel much better.

BRCA gene mutations and HER2-negative breast cancer. In normal cells, the BRCA1 and BRCA2 genes produce proteins that help repair DNA when it becomes damaged. Poly ADP-ribose polymerase (PARP) proteins also aid in fixing damaged DNA. About 7% of breast cancers are caused by mutations in the BRCA1 or BRCA2 genes. When either BRCA1 or BRCA2 is mutated in breast cancer cells, the cells cannot fix damaged DNA as well and they rely on PARP proteins to do this job. Targeted therapies called PARP inhibitors block PARP proteins, thus causing the death of these cancer cells. Olaparib and talazoparib are oral PARP inhibitors that may be used to treat HER2-negative metastatic breast cancer in people who have a mutation in BRCA1 or BRCA2. Olaparib may also be helpful to treat some patients with early-stage, HER2-negative cancer and a gene mutation in BRCA1 or BRCA2.

Antibody-drug conjugates. These drugs, also called ADCs, are made of an antibody linked to chemotherapy. The antibody part of the drug binds to something specific to breast cancer cells. The drug then enters the cancer cell where the chemotherapy is released. Unlike traditional chemotherapy, ADCs are much more targeted to breast cancer cells with less damage to normal cells. Currently, there are three ADCs approved for use in breast cancer, two in HER2-positive breast cancer (ado-trastuzumab emtansine and fam-trastuzumab deruxtecan) and one in triple-negative breast cancer (sacituzumab govitecan-hziy).

Immunotherapy

Immunotherapy refers to treatments that are designed to augment or activate immune cells to fight the cancer. One of the major breakthroughs in cancer medicine happening right now is in the area of immunotherapy and it's important to understand how these treatments work. Cancer cells escape the immune system by co-opting the normal way your cells turn off the immune system. Whenever you have an infection, like the flu, your body needs a way of turning off the immune system once everything is okay. The proteins that govern this process are called checkpoint proteins. It turns out that cancer cells express these checkpoint proteins and turn off the immune system. We have developed drugs called checkpoint inhibitors that stop cancer cells from using this mechanism.

Oncologists are using immunotherapy to treat people with triple-negative breast cancers. The immunotherapy pembrolizumab is a checkpoint inhibitor and may be used with chemotherapy to treat metastatic triple-negative breast cancer that has programmed death-ligand 1 (PD-L1) proteins on the surface of the cells. Tumors that express PD-L1 on their surface (also called PD-L1-positive) are more likely to respond to immunotherapy than tumor cells that do not have this protein. That's why the pathologist will check this in tumor samples from patients with metastatic triple-negative breast cancer. Pembrolizumab may also be used in some patients with high-risk early-stage triple-negative breast cancer in combination with neoadjuvant chemotherapy and then continued by itself following surgery.

While most people generally tolerate immunotherapy well, others may experience serious toxicity. That's because immunotherapies can activate the immune system to such a degree that it can accidentally start attacking normal tissues and organs. There are various toxicities of immunotherapies that your doctor will be checking for, such as the potential impact on your lungs, liver, intestinal tract, or endocrine system. I would advise calling your team if you are feeling poorly while being treated with immunotherapy. Many patients on treatment with standard chemotherapy do not call if they are feeling really tired or if they have diarrhea. However, if you are being treated with immunotherapy, these side effects may represent something more serious that might need further evaluation, so I recommend calling your team to check in.

Combined Therapies

Sometimes, oncologists use a combination of several types of drugs to treat cancer. For example, people might be treated with chemotherapy followed by hormonal therapy. It can often get confusing for patients and their families, but asking about which class of drugs your treatment falls into will help you keep track of the kinds of side effects you can expect. It will also help you better understand what your team is trying to accomplish.

Bone Modifying Drugs

Osteoclasts are bone cells that break down bone tissue. Osteoclast inhibitors are drugs that block these cells from breaking down bone and therefore reduce the risk of osteoporosis and fracture. In women with metastatic breast cancer and bony metastases, these drugs help to reduce the risk of having complications from bone metastases, such as fracture, compression of the spinal cord, or the need for radiation or surgery to the bone. They also help treat an elevated calcium level. Zoledronic acid (Zometa) and denosumab (Xgeva) are two drugs that are often used to treat bony metastases in breast cancer. Zoledronic acid is given intravenously, usually every three months, and denosumab is given subcutaneously every month. These drugs are generally very well tolerated.

People often ask me about the risk of having some bony breakdown in the jaw (known as osteonecrosis of the jaw, or ONJ). This is uncommon (in about 1% of people treated with this drug) but serious, and we recommend a dental evaluation prior to starting treatment with osteoclast inhibitors. We may possibly hold treatment if you need any major dental work. Some people experience a flu-like reaction for a few days after zoledronic acid, and if this happens you can premedicate with acetaminophen (Tylenol) on subsequent infusions.

In women with early-stage breast cancer, there is some research suggesting that zoledronic acid can be used as an anti-cancer treatment in women who are postmenopausal and who have undergone treatment with chemotherapy. Women may be treated with zoledronic acid every six months for three to five years.

Getting Ready for Chemotherapy

There are several questions you will want to ask your doctor about chemotherapy to help you get oriented before you start. Even if you have already started treatment, these questions will spark important conversations as well:

- What is a cycle of chemotherapy?
- How many cycles will I need before we will know how well the treatment is working?
- How long are the infusions? What will that day entail?

- What medications do I need to take before the infusion, or what medications will be given during the infusion?
- What are the common side effects for this regimen?
- What medications will I need to take to cope with side effects?
- Who do I call if I have unexpected side effects or if I need something?
- What about my fertility? (Of course, this question isn't applicable for every patient.)

What Is a Cycle of Chemotherapy?

Chemotherapy is like many medical treatments in that you will need several of them to get good results, and a standard grouping of these treatments is called a cycle. Oncologists think in terms of cycles of chemotherapy. Every type of chemotherapy has a different measurement that constitutes a cycle. For regimens that are given once a week for two weeks (14 days) followed by a week (7 days) off, one cycle of chemotherapy refers to the two weeks treatment is given. So, there are 21 days between the first day of each new cycle. For regimens that are given every other week or every three weeks, each treatment will usually be considered its own cycle. These are rough guidelines, and you should always ask your oncologist what he or she considers a cycle for your specific chemotherapy regimen.

Your doctor should be able to tell you how many treatments you will need to complete a cycle, how many cycles of treatment you will need to complete in total, and whether there are tests that will show how well the treatment is working. Your doctor is also going to be monitoring how your body reacts to chemotherapy at different points in a cycle so they can adjust the dosage for the next cycle if you experience toxicity.

What Is Toxicity?

All chemotherapy regimens cause some side effects, but your doctor is going to be checking to see whether you are developing what's called toxicity. It sounds serious, but really it means any side effect caused by the medication. Some toxicities are so mild that we hardly pay any attention to them. For instance, some drugs will cause mouth sores that last for a day or two. Other toxicities can be life threatening, and we have to follow you closely. Luckily, you don't have to worry about what these kinds of toxicities are because we are often following them by checking in with you and looking at your labs before treatment.

Certain toxicities can happen at the beginning, middle, or end of a cycle, and your doctor will be monitoring your health to check for them. If your doctor is concerned about toxicity affecting your health, he or she may decide to give you a lower dose of the chemotherapy during the next cycle. Sometimes, your doctor may decide to hold on treating you with chemotherapy for a short period of time to allow your body to recover from toxicity. Some patients try to argue with oncologists who want to reduce the dosage or postpone a treatment. You should know that lowering the dose of chemotherapy or holding chemotherapy for a week won't necessarily reduce its efficacy. Instead, the oncologist is trying to make sure that your body can tolerate the treatment.

What Is an Infusion Like?

Intravenous chemotherapies are referred to as infusions. The length of the actual infusion will be different for each regimen of chemotherapy and includes the time for any premedications or fluids you may receive. Some infusion times are relatively short, about an hour, and some can take up to five or six hours, so it's good to ask how long the infusion will take for your type of chemotherapy.

While in the infusion unit, you will be attended to by nurses who are experts at answering your questions about the process and making you more comfortable. They can get you blankets and ice chips and help keep you updated on the progress of the infusion. In some hospitals you will have the same infusion nurse throughout your treatment, and he or she will get to know you really well and be an enormous asset during this time.

In addition to administering the actual infusion, these nurses are carrying out the important function of double-checking the doses of the medications that have been ordered and checking with the pharmacy to see when they will be mixed. Infusion nurses are also communicating with your doctor about how you are doing on any given day. If you are being given extra medications or fluids through your IV to help with side effects, infusion nurses know exactly what these are and why they are being given. So if you have questions about anything, this is the person to ask. Infusion nurses also have a lot of information and tips about how to deal with side effects.

Do I Need a Portacath?

We sometimes recommend that people who are getting intravenous chemotherapy get a portacath, also called a port. These are special devices that allow access to veins and are implanted under your skin (figure 4.1). The port is a disk with a chamber that attaches to an intravenous catheter so that the infusions can be delivered into your bloodstream. This prevents the nurses from having to insert an IV line into your arm with every infusion, and it allows nurses to easily do a blood draw without searching for a vein in the arm.

A port is not merely a convenience for infusion nurses, however. Many patients hate the constant sticks in the arm that it can take to find a vein for infusions. And after several months of infusions, some of the veins can become scarred and difficult to access. Additionally, some chemotherapy drugs can be given only through a port because they are too toxic to administer through smaller peripheral veins, such as those in your arm or hand.

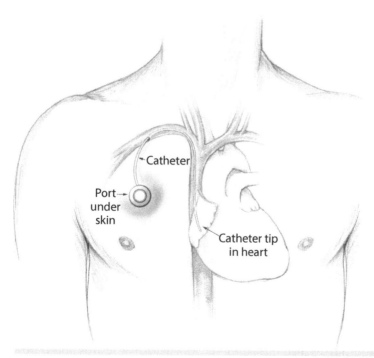

Figure 4.1. Placement of a portacath

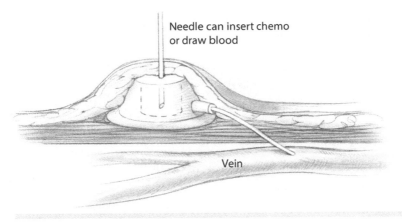

Needle can insert chemo
or draw blood

Vein

Figure 4.2. Inserting a needle into a portacath

Sometimes a port can be used the same day it is inserted. A port can be inserted prior to starting chemotherapy or after treatment has started. An interventional radiologist or surgeon at your hospital will insert the port with a procedure that generally takes about 45 minutes. You will receive local anesthesia to numb your skin along with intravenous medications to lessen any pain and anxiety. When the procedure is finished and the local anesthesia wears off, you will feel some discomfort that should resolve over the course of a day. It's fine to take acetaminophen or oxycodone for a day or two to ease the discomfort. The port will look like a half-dollar just underneath the skin below your collarbone. An infusion nurse can insert a needle into the port to give you intravenous medications or fluids, or to take a blood draw (figure 4.2). After the incision is healed, you can shower and swim.

It is important to note that there are two major concerns about ports. The first is that they can become infected, so anyone who accesses the port has to be careful to keep the area sterile. Ports can also clot, and they can be a source of blood clots that can travel to the lung. If a port becomes infected or clotted, it almost always has to be removed. Ultimately, you should ask your doctor whether a port is right for you.

What Is a Day of Chemo Like?

While the infusion itself may take only a short time, a typical day in the clinic is likely to be much longer. Like most everything associated with medical treatment, there will be several necessary steps you have to go through along with some waiting around. To get an infusion, all these steps have to happen in order:

1. A nurse or technician draws some blood so that the lab can do a complete blood count and a metabolic panel to check your liver and kidney function.

2. You meet your clinician, either your oncologist or the nurse practitioner, for a checkup.

3. The clinician checks your blood work and orders the chemotherapy to be mixed in the pharmacy.

4. You go to the infusion unit and wait for a room or chair to be available.

5. The nurse sets up your IV.

6. The chemotherapy drugs are delivered to the floor and double-checked by your nurse.

7. You get medications or fluids to prepare for chemotherapy.

8. Your nurse administers the infusion.

Sometimes the lab gets backed up doing blood counts, sometimes your clinician is running late because of an emergency, and sometimes the pharmacy gets overwhelmed with chemotherapy orders. So the infusion may not start exactly at the appointed time. People often express their anxiety about being late for their infusion appointment, and I reassure them that the nurses on the unit know that things often don't run according to schedule and are accustomed to patients coming in later than their scheduled appointment time. They know that they can't give an infusion until the blood work comes in, the clinician orders the chemo, and the lab has mixed it. In this case, it's okay to just relax and trust the process.

I find that patients do best when they plan to spend an entire day in the infusion unit by bringing something to do: a book to read, movies to watch, or a loved one or friend to spend some of the day with them. Then, if things run really smoothly and they are done more quickly than expected, they consider it a bonus. There are several other things you can do to help speed things along as well:

Get the blood work done early. If you arrive 30 to 45 minutes before your appointment time to have your blood drawn, you will have a better chance of having the labs back when you see your clinician. Then you can get right to the infusion unit.

Keep a log of what you experience after each infusion. The doctor is going to ask a lot of predictable questions about how you felt after your last infusion, how much you ate, whether you experienced nausea or other bothersome symptoms, how long you were fatigued. Having ready answers means that the doctor has the best information and can make decisions based on how your body is reacting to treatment.

Have your list of questions ready for your clinician. Your doctor will be asking you about side effects and the doses of medications you are taking to control side effects. If you have a list of questions or concerns about side effects or can detail how you felt after the previous infusion, your doctor can help you with those right away, and you won't worry that you are forgetting something. If you have questions about when you will be getting scans or how your blood work looks, this is the time to ask.

Additional Medications

After you get to the infusion unit and your nurse has the chemotherapy mixed for you in hand, you will get different medications to help with the side effects of the chemotherapy. You might get antinausea medications, like ondansetron, which are more fully explained in chapter 9. These drugs dramatically reduce the nausea that patients experience from chemotherapy. You might also have been instructed to take some steroids the night before the chemotherapy infusion. Taking all these medications as prescribed is crucial to minimize the side effects of the infusion itself.

Allergic Reactions

Many people have allergies of some kind, and most people know of someone who is allergic to some class of medication. Chemotherapy is no different in that there are some people who have, or develop, an allergic reaction to the chemotherapy drug they are being given. Rest assured that infusion nurses are experts at seeing and treating even mild allergic reactions. This is one of the reasons they will be constantly checking on you to see how you are responding to each infusion.

Most times an allergic reaction is mild, such as a single hive on your arm. It's rare but possible for certain patients to develop an overwhelming allergic reaction, called anaphylaxis, in which the tongue will begin to tingle and swell and the person may start to wheeze or cough. In some people, a reaction is preceded by a funny feeling in the head or body—and, in a few of these cases, people have a severe and sudden reaction in which they pass out before they know what's happening. Know that a capable nurse will be steps away from you at all times during your infusion and that if you do have even a mild reaction, your nurse will stop your infusion immediately and give you medications such as steroids and antihistamines to stop the reaction.

Patients who do have a severe reaction may have to see an allergist to undergo desensitization to the chemotherapy, just as you would undergo desensitization to penicillin if you were allergic and really needed it.

Side Effects

You probably already know that chemotherapy causes some side effects. The classic examples in movies and television are nausea and hair loss, but every regimen is different, and some regimens don't result in either of these. Some side effects, such as nausea, can be controlled well with medication, while most—including hair loss—are temporary. Also, side effects like nausea will change and improve in the days following an infusion, while other side effects may be cumulative over the course of a cycle of treatment.

The best way to prepare is to ask your oncologist what kinds of side effects are common for your regimen. Rather than asking for the entire list of possibilities, though, ask for a list of the top three. Ask whether these side effects happen almost always, usually, or only sometimes. Ask how long these side effects are likely to last. You will also want to know whether any of the side effects can be cumulative. Will they likely be worst during the first infusions, or are they likely to be worst during the final infusions of a cycle? Could they be permanent? Who do you call when something seems amiss or when you have a question? That last question is extremely important. Ask your team how to contact them with urgent questions if you are not feeling well, even it's after office hours. For nonurgent questions, you may have the option to send an electronic message through a patient portal.

Knowing the answers to these questions will help you plan the other activities in your life so that you are doing the things that are important to you when your energy is highest and when you feel most like yourself. Although such side effects as fatigue and nausea or rashes or mouth sores are disruptive and frustrating, there will likely be days during treatment when you feel pretty good. We talk a lot in treatment about planning to cope during those days when you feel crummy, but you also want to plan for those days when you feel strong and able to get out and live your life.

Here is a list of the most common side effects:

Fatigue. Most people experience fatigue in two ways. There is the immediate fatigue that a person feels after the infusion of chemotherapy. Some people fall asleep during the infusion. Most patients just hunker down those first couple days until they begin to feel better. The other kind of fatigue is more cumulative. If you are getting chemotherapy for several cycles, you may be more tired at the end of a cycle or at the end of several cycles. Plan to get out and move around when you feel most energetic. Even going for a short walk will help you stay energized and keep you from becoming deconditioned, which can make you even more tired. We discuss fatigue more in chapter 16.

Nausea. Some chemotherapy regimens are more or less likely to cause nausea, and the timing of nausea can also be variable. It might appear right after the infusion, or several days later. Some people feel nauseated just before the treatments, even in the car on their way to their appointment. There are really powerful drugs to help prevent or decrease this side effect of therapy, and if your chemotherapy regimen is one that is likely to cause nausea, you will be receiving some intravenous antinausea medications even before you receive your chemotherapy. Your doctor will also give you various medications to treat nausea that you might experience at home. If you experience nausea, sometimes it is helpful to steer yourself toward foods that you know you can tolerate and to eat smaller, more frequent meals.

Achiness. Some chemotherapies for breast cancer cause achiness in the muscles, joints, and bones. With some chemotherapy regimens, your doctor may also prescribe a shot that boosts the white blood cells, also known as white blood cell growth factors (pegfilgrastim is one example). It is usually administered the day after chemotherapy, and this medication can also cause achiness. Usually the symptoms go away on their own and do not limit your ability to go about your day. Occasionally, they can really be painful, and taking acetaminophen or ibuprofen may be helpful. If the achiness is thought to be caused by the white blood cell growth factor, you can ask your doctor whether she recommends trying the antihistamine loratadine for a few days, which some people find helpful.

Hair loss. Remember that not all chemotherapy causes hair loss, and you'll have to ask your doctor whether you can expect this side effect. Thinning hair typically starts to be noticeable about three weeks after the beginning of a regimen. You may notice clumps of hair in the shower or on your pillow in the morning. Some regimens cause significant (short-term) hair loss, and you may want to keep a close-cropped haircut or even be fitted for a wig near the start of your treatment. Hair loss occurs during some chemotherapy treatments and will grow back once chemotherapy is done. If you're having long term treatment for metastatic cancer, your hair may grow back with changes in your therapies. This can feel like the first of many ways in which the cancer and its treatment change your body and your sense of self. You can read more about this aspect of living with cancer in chapter 8.

With some chemotherapy regimens, your doctor may talk to you about the option of cold caps, which may help reduce hair loss. Cold cap therapy entails putting on a specially designed cap to cool the scalp during chemotherapy, thereby minimizing hair loss with some regimens. Cold cap therapy can be expensive as well as uncomfortable. And it may not be as useful for some chemotherapy regimens or for those who will be treated with more than a few cycles of chemotherapy. However, for some women, especially those undertaking certain adjuvant chemotherapy regimens (docetaxel/cyclophosphamide and paclitaxel/trastuzumab, among others), cold caps may be really effective.

Mouth sores. One common side effect of chemotherapy is the tendency to get small mouth sores for a few days after infusion. This is often called mucositis (inflammation of the mucus membrane). Some chemotherapy regimens cause irritation in the mucus membranes inside the mouth, or sometimes they activate a previous herpes infection. Rinsing with warm water mixed with baking soda and salt (1 teaspoon of each in an 8 ounce glass of water) every few hours may help with minor irritation. Mouth sores are a nuisance, although they typically heal quickly, but if they cause enough pain that you have trouble swallowing or opening your mouth or eating, you should contact your doctor.

Neuropathy. Some chemotherapies, including paclitaxel and docetaxel, can cause burning, tingling, or numbness in your fingers or toes, which may or may not be painful. These symptoms may occur for a few days after treatment and resolve by the next treatment. Or you may have symptoms that persist and affect your dexterity or balance. It may become harder to write, put on earrings, or hold your phone. Be sure to let your doctor know if you are experiencing persistent, bothersome neuropathy because the symptoms can be progressive and even permanent. Your doctor may change the dosing or schedule of your chemotherapy if you are experiencing bothersome neuropathy. For most patients who experience neuropathy, the symptoms are mild and resolve after chemotherapy has been completed.

Knowing more about the side effects of your breast cancer treatments may help you talk to your doctor about which of them you may be more or less willing to take on. I remember discussing the side effect of neuropathy with an ophthalmologist who performed delicate eye surgeries every day. When we discussed various chemotherapy options to treat her metastatic breast cancer, she opted for those with a lower chance of neuropathy given her reliance on her sense of touch to perform surgery.

Part Two of this book further details the most common ongoing side effects of treatment and how to manage them more effectively.

Planning Your Life after Infusions

Side effects tend to have a common rhythm. Many of my patients will say that they feel pretty crummy for the first two to three days immediately after the infusion. Many of them feel tired and sleep most of the first day after infusion. If the nausea is well controlled, they won't feel sick, but they won't feel like eating, either. Patients tend to feel better with each subsequent day after that until they are feeling much more like themselves. Depending on the structure of your cycle of chemotherapy, you may feel great for two weeks between infusions, or if you are on a weekly regimen, you might have only a few days that you feel like yourself.

Once you get a sense of how you are going to respond to a specific chemotherapy, you may decide a certain day is better for the infusion.

Some people like infusions early in the week so they are feeling better by the weekend, while others like the infusions later in the week so they can hunker down over the weekend and then feel better during the week. One of my patients was a special education teacher who really wanted to keep working while being treated with chemotherapy for a HER2-positive breast cancer. She didn't want to stay home the week after her infusions. She found that she preferred to get each infusion on a Friday, so that she could deal with fatigue over the weekend. By Monday, she usually felt well enough to return to teach, although she needed to cut back on tutoring after school. By the second week after each infusion, she had more energy and felt more like herself, and she occasionally would help with some after-school activities. There are no right or wrong answers. Just think about what might work best for you, and know that the clinic should be able to adapt to the schedule you prefer.

Additional Support

Starting treatment is always challenging, and cancer centers are more often including supportive services to help you relieve stress and ease into the cadence of chemotherapy. These might include massage, acupuncture, music or art therapy, or time with a social worker or religious counselor. Your palliative care team and your infusion nurses will be a great source for additional therapies available both inside the cancer clinic and within the community.

Chemo Holidays

Everybody needs a break sometimes, even in the middle of a chemotherapy regimen. You may have an important trip planned or a family gathering for which you want to feel as much like yourself as possible. Many people benefit from having a little time away from chemotherapy. You can always discuss the option of delaying a treatment to accommodate a life event or special trip. These delays are often called chemo holidays, and oncologists understand that cancer treatment is one part of your life but not your whole life. You should be able to take a break if you need one.

For those patients on lifelong chemotherapy, these breaks in treatment can be wonderful even if not tied to a specific event. Some are extended breaks from treatment that may last for several months. This will give you some time to feel normal again without having to spend time in the infusion unit. If you are receiving lifelong chemotherapy, you should definitely ask about the possibility of a chemo holiday. If you have a curable cancer with a set number of planned treatments, however, there may be excellent reasons why your doctor will not want you to take a break from chemo.

Fertility and Chemotherapy

Going through chemotherapy and other cancer therapies can affect your fertility. This can be devastating news for women who hope to have a family and may make coping with the cancer diagnosis even more challenging. Your doctors are there to help you understand this risk and the strategies you may consider to preserve your fertility. If you are hoping to get pregnant after treatment for breast cancer, it is helpful to ask your doctor a few key questions:

How serious is my diagnosis? It's important to have an open discussion with your oncologist about your prognosis and how likely it is that you may be free from cancer in the future. Additionally, your oncologist can tell you how soon you need to start chemotherapy and whether it is advisable to wait to start chemotherapy to explore options like harvesting eggs.

What is the risk that the treatment will impact my fertility? In general, women who are in their twenties and thirties are very likely to regain their periods after being treated with a time-limited course of chemotherapy given with curative intent, while women who are 40 or older are more likely to be in menopause after chemotherapy. This also depends on the chemotherapy regimen.

What are my options to preserve fertility? Your doctor may make a referral to a fertility specialist for counseling and possibly to harvest eggs prior to starting chemotherapy. During chemotherapy treatments, your doctor may discuss giving you injections to suppress your ovaries (leuprolide, for example) and put them in a temporary menopause during chemotherapy treatments. This may help increase the chance that you regain your menstrual cycle after treatment and remain fertile.

How long do I wait after chemotherapy or treatments to think about getting pregnant? While some doctors advise patients with early-stage breast cancer to wait at least two years from the diagnosis to get pregnant, there is no clear answer to this question. A discussion regarding your goals and your doctor's thoughts on safety and risk may help a person's next steps.

How Chemotherapy Affects the Family

One of the unpredictable side effects of chemotherapy is how it affects the whole family. Whether it's your spouse, children, parents, or siblings, people will react differently to your chemotherapy because they want to help but don't know how. These are incredibly stressful times for families. Everyone wants to do the right thing, but some things are more helpful than others. I am going to list some of the tricky issues that come up for patients and families. They may or may not apply to you.

- Your family is pushing your limits, thinking there is something wrong with you because you feel really tired the week you get chemotherapy. They are forever pushing you to do more than you feel you can.
- You have a mile-long list of phone calls from people who want to visit to "keep your spirits up" during treatment. You are not sure you want to see all these people when you are feeling sick.
- Your loved ones push you to eat when you are not hungry after chemotherapy and worry that you are "giving up."
- After a visit with the oncology team, everyone in your family wants an update. It is exhausting.
- Your loved ones are able to come to appointments only intermittently. When they do, they ask your doctors all kinds of questions about matters you have already discussed with them. It feels like they don't believe that you are telling about what the doctors have said.

Over the years, I have found some things help treatment go more smoothly. First, have the same one or two people come to your appointments on a consistent basis, particularly the appointments when you might be reviewing a biopsy or scan or discussing a new treatment. One of them should be your health care proxy. You need to designate a person to make medical decisions for you if you are too sick to make them yourself. It's helpful for your health care proxy to be present for all appointments where results or treatments are discussed so they hear the same information that you are hearing. It is also important to talk about your wishes for treatments with this person.

During these appointments your loved ones have the opportunity to ask as many questions as they like. You can encourage a discussion about any of the issues they have been worried about. Sometimes it is helpful for them to hear the same message from your team that you are telling them. Sometimes they will want more or less information than you want to hear. This is normal. Your spouse or your sister might want to know everything about what might happen if treatment doesn't go as well as hoped, and you may not. Or you might want to know about what might happen if the cancer progresses, while they want to hear nothing about it. Your medical team knows that you get to decide how much information you want to have about the future. And you can work with your team to get everyone's needs met.

I recently met with a patient who was on a break from chemotherapy to treat her metastatic breast cancer. Emily asked me detailed questions about what the future might bring with respect to cancer progression. Emily is a planner by nature. She likes to be prepared and she specifically wants to know how we might manage her pain as the cancer progresses and how to talk to her adult children about her prognosis. The more detail the better. Her husband, Ned, by contrast, doesn't want to talk about any of this. He only wants to know how the treatments are working now. Knowing this, we have designed our visits to include some time at the end for Emily to ask her questions while Ned waits for her in the waiting room.

You may have a larger group of people you want the oncology team to meet with as well. It is fine to talk to your oncologist about having periodic family meetings so everyone can ask their questions, and these often make sense when it is time to change to a new cancer treatment. These meetings are different from the clinic appointments that take place on the day of each infusion, however. Your infusion-day appointments become fairly routine after a while. It might be nice to have someone with you to pass the time, or it may be necessary to have someone drive you home if you are feeling crummy, but in the appointments before each infusion, your doctor will not usually be providing new information about how the treatments are working. For those appointments when your doctor will be reviewing scans or talking about treatment options, you are welcome to invite different people to join you so that everyone hears the same information at the same time.

Table 4.1. Common treatments for stage 1, 2, and 3 breast cancer

Treatment	How it is given	Common side effects	Uncommon side effects
Hormonal therapy			
Tamoxifen	Pill every day	Hot flashes, vaginal discharge, menstrual irregularity, mood changes	Blood clots, endometrial (uterine) cancer
Aromatase inhibitors (anastrozole, letrozole, exemestane)	Pill every day	Joint stiffness / achiness, hot flashes, vaginal dryness, bone density loss	Bone fracture from osteoporosis
Drugs to suppress the ovaries to put a woman into menopause (leuprolide, goserelin, triptorelin)	Monthly injection into the muscle (sometimes given every 3 months)	Hot flashes, headache, mood changes, sleep disturbances, bone density loss, discomfort at the injection site in the muscle	Bone fracture from osteoporosis
Chemotherapies			
Docetaxel / cyclophosphamide (Brand names: Taxotere / Cytoxan, so the regimen is called TC)	TC is given intravenously every 3 weeks for 4 cycles = total 12 weeks	Fatigue, nausea / vomiting, bone or muscle achiness, hair loss, fluid retention / swelling of the body, change in nails (darkened, brittle, tender), tingling / numbness in fingers / toes, low blood counts (low white blood cells, low red blood cells)	Fevers with a low white blood cell count (febrile neutropenia), inflammation of the lung (pneumonitis)

Doxorubicin/cyclophosphamide followed by paclitaxel (Brand names: Adriamycin/Cytoxan followed by Taxol, so the regimen is called AC-T)	AC is given intravenously every 2 weeks for 4 cycles, and then T is given intravenously every 2 weeks for 4 cycles or given weekly for 12 weeks. In certain situations, AC may be given every 3 weeks, and paclitaxel may be left out.	Fatigue, nausea/vomiting, hair loss, tingling/numbness in fingers/toes, bone or muscle achiness, change in urine color (orange/pink/red) for 1–2 days after treatment, low blood counts (low white blood cells, low red blood cells)	Fevers with a low white blood cell count (febrile neutropenia), inflammation of the lung (pneumonitis), leukemia, heart damage, vein irritation/injury (if given through an IV placed in the arm/hand), allergic reaction
Capecitabine	In patients with triple-negative breast cancer, if chemotherapy is given prior to surgery and there is tumor present in the surgical specimen, capecitabine pills given 2 weeks on, 1 week off for 4 to 6 months may be considered.	Fatigue, diarrhea, nausea, redness/sensitivity on the hands and soles of the feet, low blood counts (low white blood cells, low red blood cells)	Damage to the heart, including heart attacks and arrhythmias

Targeted therapy

Olaparib	May be an option for patients with a gene mutation in BRCA1 or BRCA2 and a HER2-negative cancer depending on the tumor size and lymph node involvement. Pill given twice daily for one year.	Nausea/vomiting, fatigue, headache, diarrhea, decreased appetite, decreased blood counts (white blood cells, red blood cells)	Myelodysplastic syndrome, acute myeloid leukemia, pneumonitis (a serious lung condition)

(continued)

Table 4.1 (continued)

Treatment	How it is given	Common side effects	Uncommon side effects
Chemotherapy + HER2-directed therapies			
Docetaxel/carboplatin/trastuzumab with or without pertuzumab (Brand names: Taxotere/carboplatin/Herceptin +/- Perjeta, so the regimen is called TCH or TCHP)	TCH +/- P are given intravenously every 3 weeks for 6 cycles = total of 18 weeks, and then H +/- P is given every 3 weeks to complete one year of treatment with H +/- P.	Fatigue, nausea/vomiting, hair loss, bone or muscle achiness, fluid retention/swelling of the body, tingling/numbness in fingers/toes, low blood counts (low white blood cells, low red blood cells, low platelets); additionally, with pertuzumab, diarrhea and rash may occur.	Fevers with a low white blood cell count (febrile neutropenia), inflammation of the lung (pneumonitis). Trastuzumab is generally very well tolerated with minimal to no side effects. In some cases, it may cause the heart to pump blood less effectively (congestive heart failure), which often has no symptoms and is usually not permanent.
Paclitaxel/trastuzumab (Brand names: Taxol/Herceptin, so the regimen is called TH)	TH is given intravenously every week for 12 weeks, and then H is given every 3 weeks to complete one year of treatment with H.	Fatigue, hair loss, bone or muscle achiness, tingling/numbness in fingers/toes, low blood counts (low white blood cells, low red blood cells, low platelets)	Inflammation of the lung (pneumonitis), allergic reaction, and trastuzumab side effects as listed above.
Doxorubicin/cyclophosphamide followed by paclitaxel/trastuzumab with or without pertuzumab (Brand names:	AC is given intravenously every 2 weeks for 4 cycles, and then T is given intravenously, usually weekly for 12 weeks with H +/- P given weekly or	As noted for the AC-T regimen. And with the addition of pertuzumab, diarrhea and rash may occur.	As previously noted for AC-T regimen and trastuzumab.

Adriamycin/Cytoxan followed by Taxol/Herceptin +/- Perjeta; so the regimen is called AC-TH or AC-THP)	every 3 weeks at the same time as T. After this, H +/- P is given every 3 weeks to complete one year of treatment with H +/- P.	Congestive heart failure (often with no symptoms and not permanent), allergic reaction, interstitial lung disease/pneumonitis (a serious lung condition)
Ado-trastuzumab emtansine (T-DM1)	If chemotherapy is given prior to surgery and there is tumor present in the surgical specimen, T-DM1 may be given intravenously every 3 weeks to complete one year of treatment.	Nausea, fatigue, diarrhea, low blood counts (particularly low platelets), increased liver function tests, tingling/numbness in fingers/toes
Neratinib	Neratinib may be considered after a year of adjuvant trastuzumab, particularly in tumors that were estrogen receptor-positive. There are no data evaluating neratinib after treatment with trastuzumab and pertuzumab.	Diarrhea, nausea/vomiting, abdominal pain, fatigue, skin rash, mouth ulcerations, increased liver function tests. Severe diarrhea resulting in dehydration may occur. Antidiarrheal drugs are recommended at the start of therapy with close monitoring for diarrhea.

Table 4.2. Common treatments for metastatic (stage 4) breast cancer

Hormone receptor-positive / HER2-negative breast cancer: In general, your doctor may use one of the following hormonal therapy regimens to treat metastatic breast cancer. When the tumor progresses, your doctor may select a different hormonal therapy regimen. At some point when the tumor does not seem to be responding to hormonal therapy, your doctor may switch to chemotherapy (see the treatment options under HER2-negative breast cancer later in this table). If you are premenopausal: Drugs to suppress the ovaries to put a woman into menopause (such as leuprolide) are used in addition to the treatments noted (see table 4.1 for side effects of leuprolide).

Treatment	Notes on effects
Aromatase inhibitors (anastrozole, letrozole, exemestane) + CDK4/6 inhibitors (palbociclib, abemaciclib, ribociclib)	See table 4.1 for the side effects of the aromatase inhibitors. The CDK4/6 inhibitors are pills that may cause low white blood cells, fatigue, nausea, hair thinning, diarrhea, and elevated liver function tests.
Fulvestrant + aromatase inhibitors (anastrozole, letrozole)	Fulvestrant is an injection that is given into a muscle. This injection may be uncomfortable, and the drug may cause hot flashes and joint aches.
Fulvestrant + CDK4/6 inhibitors (palbociclib, abemaciclib, ribociclib)	See side effects for each listed above.
Fulvestrant + alpelisib	Alpelisib can be added to fulvestrant for patients who have tumors that have a PIK3CA mutation. In addition to the fulvestrant side effects listed above, alpelisib may cause diarrhea, elevated blood sugars, nausea, and rash.
Everolimus + hormonal therapy (e.g., exemestane, fulvestrant, or tamoxifen)	Everolimus is a pill that is added to hormonal therapies. It may cause mouth sores, rash, fatigue, cough, swelling, high blood sugar, and diarrhea.

Treatment	Notes on effects
Fulvestrant	Fulvestrant may be used on its own. See side effects listed above.
Aromatase inhibitors (anastrozole, letrozole, exemestane)	The aromatase inhibitors may also be used on their own. See table 4.1 for the side effects of the aromatase inhibitors.
Tamoxifen	See table 4.1 for side effects of tamoxifen.
Abemaciclib	See side effects for CDK4/6 inhibitors above.

HER2-positive breast cancer: *Chemotherapy along with HER2-blocking medications are usually used first. If a tumor is also hormone receptor–positive, hormonal therapy and HER2-blocking medications may be used.*

Treatment	Notes on effects
Docetaxel or paclitaxel + trastuzumab + pertuzumab	Trastuzumab and pertuzumab are HER2-blocking medications that are given in intravenous or subcutaneous formulations (toxicities in table 4.1).
Ado-trastuzumab emtansine (T-DM1)	T-DM1 is chemotherapy linked to trastuzumab. The main side effects are listed in table 4.1.
Fam-trastuzumab deruxtecan	Trastuzumab deruxtecan is also chemotherapy linked to trastuzumab. The main side effects are fatigue, nausea/vomiting, hair loss, and constipation. Interstitial lung disease/pneumonitis (a serious lung condition) can occur.
Tucatinib + trastuzumab + capecitabine	Tucatinib is a pill that blocks HER2. Tucatinib may cause diarrhea, redness/sensitivity on the hands and soles of the feet, nausea, fatigue, and increased liver function tests. (The side effects of capecitabine and trastuzumab are listed in table 4.1.)
Trastuzumab + chemotherapy (various options)	

(continued)

Table 4.2 (continued)

Treatment	Notes on effects
Capecitabine + trastuzumab or lapatinib	Lapatinib is a pill that blocks HER2. Lapatinib may cause a rash, diarrhea, mouth sores, fatigue, and nausea. (The side effects of capecitabine and trastuzumab are listed in table 4.1.)
Trastuzumab + lapatinib	See above.
Neratinib + capecitabine	Neratinib is a pill that blocks HER2. The toxicities of neratinib and capecitabine are listed in table 4.1.
Margetuximab + chemotherapy (capecitabine, eribulin, gemcitabine, or vinorelbine)	Margetuximab is a HER2-blocking medication given intravenously along with chemotherapy.
For HER2-positive breast cancers that are also estrogen receptor–positive or progesterone receptor–positive, the treatment options for those who are postmenopausal (or being treated with ovarian suppression) are as follows: Aromatase inhibitor +/− trastuzumab Aromatase inhibitor +/− lapatinib Aromatase inhibitor +/− lapatinib + trastuzumab Fulvestrant +/− trastuzumab Tamoxifen +/− trastuzumab	See table 4.1 for side effects.

HER2-negative breast cancer: *Usually one chemotherapy is used at a time, although sometimes a combination of chemotherapies might be used at the same time. There is no recommendation for one specific chemotherapy over another, and chemotherapy selection is individualized based on prior treatment, patient's overall health, tumor characteristics, and side effects. Most chemotherapies, including those listed in this table, can cause fatigue, lowering of blood counts, nausea, appetite or taste changes, and mouth sores. Talk to your oncology team about side effects to anticipate and review the most common ones on pages 54–57 of the main text. Unless specified for use with triple-negative breast cancer, these therapies can be used to treat hormone receptor–positive breast cancer, usually after it has progressed on hormonal therapy.*

Doxorubicin	See table 4.1

Liposomal doxorubicin	Does not usually cause total hair loss.
Paclitaxel	See table 4.1.
Capecitabine	Capecitabine is the one chemotherapy for metastatic breast cancer that is given in pill form (toxicities in table 4.1). Does not usually cause total hair loss.
Gemcitabine	Does not usually cause total hair loss.
Vinorelbine	May cause neuropathy, constipation. Does not usually cause total hair loss.
Eribulin	May cause neuropathy.
Sacituzumab govitecan-hziy (for triple-negative breast cancer)	Sacituzumab is a Trop2-directed antibody linked to chemotherapy. It may cause decreased blood counts (white blood cells, red blood cells), diarrhea, nausea/vomiting, fatigue, and an allergic reaction.
Cisplatin or carboplatin (for triple-negative breast cancer and in people with a BRCA1/2 mutation)	May cause neuropathy; do not usually cause total hair loss.
Pembrolizumab + chemotherapy (for PD-L1-positive, triple-negative breast cancer: chemotherapy options include albumin-bound paclitaxel, or paclitaxel, or gemcitabine plus carboplatin)	Pembrolizumab is immunotherapy. It is generally well tolerated but there are serious and potentially life-threatening side effects that the oncology team monitors (inflammation of the lung, colon, liver, or heart; problems with the pituitary or thyroid gland).
Olaparib and talazoparib (nonchemotherapy options for HER2-negative patients with a mutation in the BRCA1 or BRCA2 gene as well)	Both olaparib and talazoparib are PARP inhibitors given in pill form. They may cause nausea/vomiting, fatigue, diarrhea, headache, decreased appetite, decreased blood counts (white blood cells, red blood cells, platelets), and/or elevated liver function tests. There are higher rates of hair loss reported with talazoparib (25%) when compared to olaparib (3%).
Cyclophosphamide	As noted for AC-T regimen in table 4.1.
Docetaxel	As noted for TC and TCH regimens in table 4.1.
Albumin-bound paclitaxel	May cause neuropathy, allergic reactions.

CHAPTER FIVE

Tests and Scans in Treatment

If you are undergoing chemotherapy to treat breast cancer, you may have heard that there are a lot of routine blood tests to see how well your body is tolerating the treatment. Patients at any stage of breast cancer who are being treated with chemotherapy will, in fact, need regular blood tests to make sure that the oncologist can safely give chemotherapy. This chapter describes the different blood tests your doctor will be looking at and what the results might mean.

Patients with metastatic breast cancer will also need regular scans to see how the tumors are responding to treatment. For some women, there are also genomic and genetic tests that may provide more information about the cancer or the risk of getting another cancer. This data may guide your doctor's breast cancer screening and treatment recommendations. The results may cause significant changes in your treatment regimen, and if you know why these various tests are done and what the results mean, you can better understand what's happening in your body and what your medical team is telling you.

All that said, not every patient will need tests. Breast cancer is different from other types of cancer in that many patients don't need routine scans and blood work. This can be confusing because many patients expect treatment to be followed by blood testing and imaging studies. The need for tests and scans really depends on the stage of your cancer and what cancer therapies are being used. For example, a person with early-stage hormone receptor–positive breast cancer who underwent a lumpectomy, radiation, and hormonal therapy may only need annual mammograms to make sure the cancer has not returned. So let's walk through the possibilities.

Blood Tests

Blood tests are going to be a big part of your life if you are being treated with chemotherapy for either early-stage breast cancer or metastatic breast cancer. Patients undergoing chemotherapy need to have their blood drawn every time they come to the clinic for treatment, and there are three main categories of blood tests that your oncologist may order: blood counts, chemistries, and tumor markers.

You might hate the idea of having blood taken, and neither Vicki, Dave, nor I blame you. While many nurses and technicians are experts at finding a vein and slipping the needle in painlessly, not everyone can do this every time. If you've had a portacath placed under your skin for infusions, you should ask the nurse to do the blood draws through that instead of your skin. It may take a few minutes to have this nurse put a needle into your port, but it is usually less painful than getting a needle stick. Also, there are creams that contain such local anesthetics as lidocaine and prilocaine that can be applied to the skin above your port site that make accessing your port more comfortable. You can ask your oncology team to prescribe this for you if you experience pain when the port is accessed.

Blood Counts

A complete blood count (CBC) measures the three main types of blood cells that your bone marrow makes:

White blood cells. This is the army of immune soldiers that fight infection in your system. When your white blood count is low, you are prone to serious infection and can rapidly get very sick without knowing it.

Red blood cells. These carry oxygen around your body. When the red blood count is low, you have anemia. If you are very anemic, you may experience fatigue and breathlessness.

Platelets. These help the blood to clot, and if you have a low platelet count, you are more prone to bleeding, including internal bleeding.

White Blood Cells

There are two broad categories of white blood cells: myeloid cells and lymphocytes. Counting the myeloid cells is crucial because these are the ones that fight off bacteria, something your body is doing all day, every day. You may know already that you have bacteria all over your body—and that not all bacteria are bad. Your skin, respiratory tract, and gastrointestinal (GI) tract all have bacteria living in and on them as part of their natural design. Your blood cells know how to keep bacteria in check, and there is a specific subcategory of myeloid cell—called a neutrophil—that is the first line of defense against bacterial invaders in the body. Neutrophils keep bacteria at the proper level and keep them from entering the bloodstream.

You need a lot of neutrophils to stay healthy and alive. If your absolute neutrophil count (ANC) goes below 1,000, you are considered neutropenic and are at risk for developing bacteria in the bloodstream. And if bacteria do get into the bloodstream—known as sepsis, or bacteremia—you can get very sick, often over a matter of hours and sometimes with minimal symptoms. So if you are being treated with medications that may cause neutropenia, your oncology team will advise you to call if you develop a temperature above 100.4 degrees Fahrenheit. Even a slight fever is an indication that your body may be developing a life-threatening infection. It's critical that you call your cancer team for instructions on what to do next, and you may be admitted to hospital for intravenous antibiotics as your team checks in your lungs, urine, and blood for a source of infection.

A few months ago, I was paged by a young patient undergoing chemotherapy for triple-negative breast cancer. Melanie reported a temperature of 100.5 and said she felt only slightly warm but otherwise completely fine. Although I don't like referring patients to the emergency room, it is the right thing to do if a patient might have an infection. Melanie was found to have *E. coli* growing in her urine and her blood stream, along with a neutrophil count that was close to zero. Thankfully, she started antibiotics right away and was discharged from the hospital within the week. Although testing revealed the source of Melanie's infection, it is more common to find no source of infection in people with neutropenic fevers. In these situations, doctors treat with antibiotics until the neutrophil count rises to a normal range, and then they either stop antibiotics or occasionally prescribe a short course of additional antibiotics covering what is felt to be a possible source of infection.

Your CBC will report the number of neutrophils first, as a percentage of your total white blood cells (for example, 25% of 2,000), and most lab slips will do the work for you and multiply the percentage by the total white blood cells and give you the ANC (500 in this example). Oncologists keep a close eye on the ANC because we can't safely give chemotherapy unless the ANC is at a certain level—usually above 1,000. There are also other breast cancer therapies, such as the CDK4/6 inhibitors, that can lower the ANC. Your doctor will follow your CBCs regularly if you are taking these drugs.

If your doctor is concerned about your ANC dropping while you are being treated with chemotherapy, he or she may suggest something called growth factor support. Growth factors are naturally occurring proteins that your body uses to boost cell count. Drug companies have figured out how to make these growth factors (filgrastim and pegfilgrastim are two common ones), and your doctor can administer them to you after you get chemotherapy.

Your CBC will also contain a count for the second type of white blood cell, called a lymphocyte. These are the generals of the immune system because they direct all the other white blood cells in attacking an infection. While they are less important than neutrophils on a day-to-day basis, they are the core of your immune system. (For example, a T cell, which is attacked in HIV infections, is a type of lymphocyte.) The good news is that most chemotherapy drugs don't affect the lymphocytes to a significant degree. However, people with low- or poor-functioning lymphocytes are susceptible to so-called opportunistic infections, which are those caused by uncommon bacteria or viruses. Patients may get opportunistic infections when they are on steroids (such as prednisone and dexamethasone) for long periods of time (as in cases of managing a tumor in the brain or spinal cord), if they are being treated for inflammation in their lungs from radiation or chemotherapy, or if they are experiencing a serious side effect from immunotherapy. In these scenarios, steroids can decrease the effectiveness of lymphocytes and put people at risk for opportunistic infections. So if you are prescribed steroids for more than a month, your doctor may also prescribe an antibiotic like trimethoprim-sulfamethoxazole (Bactrim) to try to prevent these infections from happening.

Red Blood Cells

Your oncologist is going to be watching your blood work for anemia, too, as cancer itself and cancer therapies such as chemotherapy can inhibit your bone marrow's ability to make red blood cells. If cancer is the cause, we call it anemia of chronic disease, and if chemotherapy is the cause, we call it chemotherapy-induced anemia. Radiation can also cause anemia by damaging your bone marrow, and some women may also be anemic from heavy menstruation. In rare cases, anemia can develop from other blood loss, such as bleeding from a tumor that is infiltrating healthy tissue. Patients with metastatic breast cancer who have been on several chemotherapies are more prone to anemia because the bone marrow has a harder time producing blood cells after so much exposure to chemotherapy. Sometimes, breast cancer infiltrates bone marrow and takes up space, leading to less production of blood cells in general.

If you have anemia, you may experience fatigue or shortness of breath. Each person is different and some don't experience symptoms even when their red blood cell count is very low. It's also often hard to know if a symptom like fatigue is from anemia, from the cancer therapies, or from being less active than normal. You probably won't have any symptoms from anemia unless your red blood count, or hematocrit, falls below 30. If you are symptomatic from anemia or if your hematocrit is very low (at a level of 21, with or without symptoms), your doctor may recommend a blood transfusion.

Blood Chemistries

After counting the number and type of cells in your blood sample, the lab will test for chemical compounds found in your blood. We call these results the blood chemistries, and there are three results your doctor will be looking at: electrolytes, kidney function, and liver function. These tests should be ordered for you at every visit to the clinic in which you get an infusion, and the lab will need about 45 minutes to return the results. If you are being treated with chemotherapy and these numbers are abnormal, your doctor will have to assess whether it is safe to treat you that day. You should expect to arrive at the clinic at least 45 minutes before your scheduled infusion to get your blood drawn and your labs started.

Electrolytes are minerals in your system, and they are often part of a blood screening because they are markers of health, such as the proper balance of hydration, and an electrolyte imbalance can be an early sign of a developing problem. Your oncologist will be looking at your levels of sodium, potassium, magnesium, and calcium. When these are too high or too low, doctors know to look further, because you might be sick without realizing it.

Kidney (or renal) function is a critical marker for your doctor to monitor during treatment as well. Many of the drugs that you take are filtered out over time and eliminated by the kidneys. If your kidneys aren't functioning well to filter your blood, certain medications can accumulate in the bloodstream and become toxic. This is particularly true of chemotherapy drugs and the bisphosphonates, such as zoledronic acid (also known as Zometa). Kidney function tests include the blood urea nitrogen and the creatinine. Usually your blood urea nitrogen is less than 20 milligrams per deciliter and your creatinine is less than 1 milligram per deciliter.

If these are abnormal, your doctor will look into it right away and may even delay your next infusion. Many times there is an easy explanation for abnormal kidney function. It could be something as simple as dehydration caused by one of the chemotherapy drugs. Whatever the reason, your oncologist will be paying close attention to these numbers.

In addition to electrolytes and kidney function, your doctor will be looking at your liver function tests (LFT). You may already know that the liver carries out the vital function of clearing the blood of toxins, but it also makes many of the necessary proteins for the body. These proteins are created in the hepatocytes, the main cells of the liver. If those cells are damaged, they will release enzymes into the blood that can be measured in the lab. So your doctor is going to be looking at something called aspartate aminotransferase (AST) and alanine aminotransferase (ALT). When these numbers go up, doctors usually suspect inflammation of the liver caused by chemotherapy drugs. An elevated level can also mean that there are cancer cells active in the liver.

What you need to know is that your doctor may be reluctant to give more cancer therapy in the short term when AST or ALT levels go up. He or she may be concerned that your liver cells won't be able to effectively filter the drug out of your system, which means you would be at risk for developing toxic levels of the drug in your blood. I have a patient with a history of metastatic breast cancer being treated with letrozole and ribociclib. She came to see me feeling great, but her labs showed that her LFTs had shot up. Since this is a known side effect of the ribociclib, we temporarily stopped the drug. She stayed on letrozole and we monitored her LFTs until they normalized. Then we were able to restart ribociclib at a lower dose without any further liver issues.

Your liver also makes bile that gets secreted through the biliary tree and into the small intestine. An elevated alkaline phosphatase (ALP, or alk phos) level reveals damage to cells near the bile ducts. Bilirubin is actually a yellowish substance in the bile, and if the duct is blocked, that substance will build up in your bloodstream. When you have way too much of it in your system, your skin and the whites of your eyes will actually turn yellow. Many breast cancer therapies, including chemotherapy and the CDK4/6 inhibitors, are also eliminated through the biliary system, and so your doctor will want to investigate any elevated levels of ALP and bilirubin. You may be asked to get an abdominal ultrasound or a CT scan looking for dilated bile ducts, which would indicate that something is blocking the ducts.

Tumor Markers

Cancer cells are constantly producing proteins that get secreted into the bloodstream. Lab technicians can measure the levels of some of these proteins, and the result is what we call tumor markers. In general, the more cancer cells you have, the higher the tumor markers in your blood. As the number of cancer cells decreases, the marker numbers go down.

In patients being treated for an early-stage breast cancer, we don't check tumor markers because it does not lead to improved cure rates or survival. If you have a friend with colon cancer, you may know that tumor markers are often followed in early-stage cancer, and an elevated tumor marker may prompt more testing that may lead to interventions such as surgery. This is not true for early-stage breast cancer. We do consider checking tumor markers in people with metastatic cancer, though, because they can sometimes give us a way to monitor the cancer and its response to therapy between scans. Some common tumor markers checked in breast cancer are CA 15-3, CA 27-29, and CEA (carcinoembryonic antigen).

The whole subject of tumor markers can be confusing. First, not all tumors produce tumor markers, so your tumor markers may be in the normal range even before you start treatment. In this case, we know the tumor markers are completely uninformative, and we don't usually check them again. Second, not all cancers with the same markers produce the same level of that marker. So you can't compare your tumor marker to your neighbor's. Your tumor markers are specific to your cancer alone. Third, even normal tissues can produce these markers, so the tumor markers may be more elevated for reasons other than cancer. At this point, you may be wondering why doctors bother to follow these numbers at all.

If you have metastatic cancer, meaning you have tumors in multiple sites of your body, your doctor may monitor the tumor markers to see how treatment is working. When those levels go down over time, we suspect that the tumors are getting smaller or that there are fewer cancerous cells circulating in your body. While the reduction of tumor markers is a great sign, your doctor will always order scans to confirm the result. Overall, you can think of tumor markers as providing some extra information about whether your tumor might be responding to cancer therapies in between scans.

I have patients who are engineers and teachers, and they sometimes make charts or spreadsheets of their blood work. These charts often show weekly fluctuations in tumor markers, which can cause distress when the tumor markers are up a little from a prior measurement. Unfortunately, tumor markers do change week to week—even day to day—but those small changes don't actually signal anything. Cells generate more or less of these proteins based on many factors. Tumor markers correlate only generally to the tumor burden in your body and aren't a specific measurement of the tumors themselves.

Scans or No Scans?

Before I review the types of scans you might receive in treatment, it's worth talking about why you might not need routine scans at all while in treatment for early-stage breast cancer. Oncologists generally do not recommend routine imaging studies (apart from regular mammograms) in women treated for early-stage breast cancer because they have not been shown to help women live longer. This can be confusing. Often, a patient will ask me why she is not having routine CT scans or PET scans to check for the possibility that the cancer has spread. Because we've all been told that routine screening and early diagnosis of breast cancer can improve survival, it's natural to assume that this logic would extend to identifying metastases early. But it's not that simple.

Imagine a woman being treated for early-stage cancer who has no symptoms of progressing cancer. If she had a scan that showed metastases, this would change her diagnosis from early-stage to metastatic. And she would probably start a cancer therapy at this time. If this same woman had no scan until two or three months later when she presented to her doctor with a symptom like pain, her prognosis would be the same. Her life expectancy in both scenarios would be exactly the same. Breast cancers often respond well to treatment, so finding additional tumors a few months early doesn't change their response to treatment.

That doesn't mean that women with early-stage breast cancer never have scans ordered for them. If you have a symptom that bothers you and persists over time, you should discuss it with your medical team. I encourage my patients to call me with any symptom that sticks around for more than two weeks so I can do the thinking and worrying about whether this is cancer-related. I will usually see the person in clinic to get more details and to examine her, and if there is a concern that the symptom may be caused by cancer, we can order imaging to check it out.

Ask anyone about life with metastatic breast cancer, on the other hand, and inevitably the conversation will come around to scans. This is the primary way you and your doctor will follow your progress and see how your treatment is working. Specifically, scans are radiology studies that image your body. They include computed tomography (CT), positron emission tomography (PET), bone scan, and magnetic resonance imaging (MRI).

If you are in treatment for metastatic breast cancer, you will likely have scans every few months, and you will usually review those scans with your doctor a day or two after they have been taken. Waiting for scan results can be distressing, and you want to shorten your wait as much as possible. Make sure you schedule an appointment with your oncologist first, and then schedule the scan for a day or so before. That way you minimize your wait time, and you know that when you see your oncologist the scans will be ready and you can look at them and talk about them together.

If you have a patient portal, your scan results may be available to you before you see your oncologist. Many people express anxiety about reading these results on their own before they review them with their oncologist. If this is the case, try your best to wait. Some of my patients find it helpful to turn off the alert on their phones that notify them of new test results.

Some patients ask to go over the scans by phone. I almost always insist that they come into the clinic. The phone is not ideal for these conversations, and it is so easy to miscommunicate about really important aspects of your care. It's usually best to review scans face-to-face. These visits can be some of the most meaningful and important conversations you have with your oncologist because they often lead to detailed discussions about prognosis and treatment. I always recommend bringing someone from your support team with you to take notes and remember what went on during the discussion after you have left the office.

Also, you can ask your oncologist if they've reviewed your scans with the radiologist. Scans are tricky to interpret, and if your oncologist is just reading the radiologist's report, he or she may have missed some of the subtleties. Your doctor knows everything about how you are feeling, and the radiologist knows everything about what the scans say. So, if there is any question about the significance of a finding on your scan, it's important that your doctor talk to the radiologist. This conversation is the chance for your doctor to ask important follow-up questions about what the radiologist has seen.

I am treating a young woman with metastatic breast cancer who has had an exceptional response to chemotherapy. Prior to treatment, she had significant liver metastases. Because of a tumor in her hip, she was unable to walk and needed high doses of opioids to control her pain. Once she started chemotherapy, she felt better overall and started eating and gaining weight. Within two weeks, one of her tumor markers had dropped by 90%. A few weeks later, she was off of opioids and walking slowly with the help of physical therapy. These were all good signs that treatment was working well. So, I was shocked when her scan report indicated that the tumors in her liver were getting larger and that her disease was progressing. I went to the reading room to sit beside one of the radiologists and see her imaging myself. After they heard more about how she was doing, they reviewed her scans and noticed that while the liver tumors were larger, the increased size was due to necrosis, or dying tumor cells, within the tumors. This was caused by the dramatic response to treatment.

CT Scans

Computerized tomography are the most common scans ordered by doctors. The scans take thousands of pictures of your body in slices, and then sophisticated software reconstructs those slices into a three-dimensional whole. You may have had one of these scans during the process of staging your cancer, and the subsequent scans will be similar.

Contrasts

A CT scan is most helpful in tracking cancer when there is some kind of contrast in the body, a substance that helps highlight blood vessels and makes more tumors visible (since they are often more vascular than the surrounding tissue). Patients getting a scan of the abdomen may be asked to take an oral contrast, something you drink before the scan that outlines the GI tract and makes it easier to distinguish from other tissues. The oral contrast may cause some cramping and diarrhea, and if it does, you should stop taking it. And the truth is, oral contrast isn't critical to reading most scans. IV contrast, however, is usually important, and it should be given in most instances. With intravenous contrast, doctors can more easily see tumors because it will help outline the areas of cancer on the scan.

The problem with IV contrast is that some people begin to develop allergies to it, and if that happens, doctors worry that it can lead to anaphylactic shock. You'll know you are developing an allergy if you get an itchy feeling after the IV starts or develop hives on your skin. In that case, we may have to administer steroids before the IV contrast. Sometimes the steroids are effective in controlling the allergy, but sometimes people simply can't tolerate the IV contrast even with the steroids and it needs to be omitted altogether. The IV contrast may also not be appropriate for people with poor kidney function because it can lead to kidney failure. These are some reasons your doctor may omit either or both contrasts before your scan.

Reading CT Scans

When you look at a CT scan, the different images may not look like much of anything to you, but your doctor can point out the bones and different organs and can scroll through each slice to show you the outlines of visible tumors. A tumor needs to be about 5 millimeters in size to be visible. If it is any smaller, it will blend into the surrounding tissue. Yet that tiny 5-millimeter tumor will still contain about 1 billion cancer cells. People are astounded to learn that they can have a collection of 100 million cancer cells in a tumor that is still too small to detect on a scan. That's why doctors follow scans over time when treating a patient with metastatic cancer. This is the only way we can see whether something is growing or shrinking.

Doctors use all kinds of terms to describe cancer: nodule, mass, tumor, lesion. It's easy to get hung up on these words, but they all mean cancer. Sometimes it's easy to follow the progress of cancer with CT scans: a lemon-sized lesion can become orange sized, or it can shrink down to the size of a walnut. If progress is slower, we can still put calipers around lesions and measure them accurately. But it's not always so straightforward. Some cancer spreads less like a discrete mass and more like a moss that grows along the planes of a tissue, making it difficult to tell the normal tissue from the cancer. Peritoneal carcinomatosis, which grows in the abdomen, has spreads more like grains of sand, and this can be hard to quantify and track in a CT scan.

PET Scans

Positron emission tomography scans are nuclear medicine scans. A radiologist injects a radioactive isotope into the veins and then can detect where that substance accumulates. For a PET scan, radiologists usually use something called fluorodeoxyglucose, which is a glucose-based dye that is taken up readily by metabolically active tissues such as cancer.

PET scans don't give good spatial resolution so they are often combined with a CT scan, and these scans are called PET-CTs. The CT portion of a PET-CT is often a noncontrast CT with nondiagnostic quality. The CT is just good enough for us to be able to note where the fluorodeoxyglucose is being accumulated. Your oncologist can ask for a diagnostic quality CT scan to be merged to a PET scan, too, which may provide more information.

Patients will often insist that they get PET scans because they think that PET scans are better than CT scans. But that's not usually the case in breast cancer since breast cancer cells are generally not as metabolically active as other types of cancer cells. Since they are less metabolically active, they don't take up as much of the glucose-based dye, meaning the PET scan may not show a cancer that may be there. In general, national cancer guidelines recommend following patients with metastatic cancer with CT scans and bone scans, and this is what I do in my practice. Sometimes, it may be hard to tell if a lesion on a CT scan is cancer, and I may consider checking a PET-CT scan to see if it adds any additional information.

Bone Scans

A bone scan is another type of nuclear medicine scan that your doctor might order if they suspect that your cancer has metastasized to the bones. For this test, you will have a very small amount of radioactive material injected into your veins. After a two- to four-hour wait, you will come back for a scan. The radioactive material will usually collect within the bone in areas where there are metastases. However, a bone scan is not specific to cancer and will also show areas of fracture, arthritis, or infection.

MRI Scans

An MRI uses magnetic fields and radio waves to form images of the body. The radiologist may also use a contrast agent called gadolinium, which is generally safe unless you have poor kidney function. These tests are much better than CT scans at imaging a particular organ. In patients with metastatic breast cancer, the most common reasons for getting an MRI is to get an image of the brain, spinal cord, and liver because the MRI does a better job of finding metastases in these areas. As a patient, though, you may prefer a CT scan, because the MRI requires you to lay inside a large tube and hold still for up to an hour. It can also be loud inside the tube. All of this combined can be distressing if you suffer from claustrophobia or have trouble holding one position because of pain. You can take antianxiety medication, such as lorazepam, or pain medication, such as morphine, before getting an MRI.

Scan Results

In general, there are only three results that any of these scans will show while you are in treatment for metastatic cancer. First, a scan could show that the cancer is responding to treatment and the tumors are getting smaller. Second, the scan could show that things are basically the same, which means that the cancer is still responding to treatment. Lastly, the scan can show that the cancer is advancing.

If your cancer is shrinking or stable, your treatments are probably doing their jobs. Sometimes my patients will be worried that the treatments are not working if the disease is stable, but I remind folks that cancer, by definition, is cells that are growing out of control. If the treatments are keeping that out-of-control growth in check, they are working well. Your doctor, then, will generally be concerned most about the third possibility: that the cancer is progressing. If your cancer is progressing, your oncologist will discuss whether it may be time to stop your current treatment and what additional treatments might be beneficial.

Unfortunately, sometimes doctors aren't sure whether things are better, worse, or the same, which can be extremely unnerving. We all want definitive news. Doctors want to be able to tell patients exactly what's going on and how well the treatment is working, and it's so easy for doctors and patients alike to feel frustrated by all the uncertainty. Remember that a scan can read a tumor only if that tumor is at least 0.5 centimeters wide, so it's possible that your body contains tumors the scan can't yet read. A scan can also show something that looks like a tumor but isn't.

In women with early-stage breast cancer who had staging CT scans at diagnosis, one of the most common causes of uncertainty are little spots on the lung called pulmonary nodules. They are too small to biopsy and too small to really identify. Nodules are common and often benign, but in patients with a history of cancer we want to make sure that it is not a metastasis. We can follow these nodules on scan after scan, and they usually don't grow or change, but sometimes they do. In fact, there are many findings on scans that are mostly likely benign but that we are obligated to follow once we find them.

Sometimes, patients and doctors worry that the radiation exposure from all the scans will put them at risk to develop more cancer. Each CT scan of the chest or abdomen gives you the same amount of radiation that you receive from general background radiation over the course of two to three years. Over many years, too much exposure to radiation can raise your risk of developing certain kinds of cancers, particularly cancers of the bone marrow, like leukemia and myelodysplastic syndrome. Usually the risk of not following one of these small, indeterminate nodules is greater than the theoretically minute risk of getting a radiation-induced cancer.

Genomic Testing

I described the use of genomic profiling of early-stage, hormone receptor–positive tumors with the use of the Oncotype DX test in chapter 2. If you have metastatic cancer, your doctor may speak with you about sending your blood and tumor tissue for additional genomic testing. One such test is called a liquid biopsy, which refers to analyzing a blood sample to look at any tumor cells it may contain. The lab will look at those tumor cells or DNA from those tumor cells to see if they contain mutations that might be responsive to specific therapies. For example, liquid tumor testing is recommended to check for PIK3CA mutation in people with hormone receptor–positive, HER2-negative metastatic breast cancer where the drug alpelisib is being considered. Alpelisib is only approved for use in those with a PIK3CA mutation, and it is used in combination with fulvestrant. The results of these tests, therefore, can guide your treatment recommendations.

Genetic Testing

Your oncologist may want you to undergo tests on your DNA, or your genetics, in part to see whether your cancer has a genetic basis and therefore runs the risk of being carried by other members of your family. This information may also provide useful information to your medical team about breast cancer screening and treatment.

Cancer is a disease of the genes, or DNA, and it develops because of an accumulation of mutations in the DNA. I like to use the illustration that a cancer cell is like a runaway train. It may run rampant because the accelerator is stuck and has overcome the braking mechanism of the train. Or the braking mechanism is faulty, so the train can't slow down or stop when it needs to. Perhaps the mechanic is incompetent and eventually the accelerating mechanism and braking mechanisms come into disrepair during normal cell division. Most cancers are due to accumulated mutations in the accelerator, braking, or mechanical parts of the genome.

The genes that you are born with are called your germline genes. Mutations occur in your germline genes that you inherited from your mom (egg) or dad (sperm). Mutations also occur in your germline genes de novo, meaning that your mom or dad didn't have them, but they occurred in the formation of the egg or sperm. Either way, some of these mutations can put you at risk for developing cancer at a young age. Genetic tests are different from the molecular pathology tests that look at the mutations specific to your cancer and driving the cancer through the malignant process. We call the latter somatic mutations to distinguish them from germline mutations.

Inherited forms of cancer are due to inherited mutations in the germline DNA that are in accelerator genes, braking genes, or the genes responsible for repairing mistakes during cell division. One of the most common inherited germline mutations are the BRCA (pronounced "bracka") mutations that put women at risk for breast and ovarian cancer. There are two main types of mutations, called BRCA1 and BRCA2, that carry different risks for different cancers. The BRCA genes are called tumor-suppressor genes and are part of that braking mechanism that the cell uses. Women who have BRCA mutations are at risk for cancers in both breasts and their ovaries. In addition, BRCA mutations also cause an increased risk for other cancers, such as pancreatic cancer, colon cancer, and prostate cancer. So if we diagnose a young woman with a BRCA gene mutation, this will not only affect her risk of developing new cancer but also the potential risk of her sisters, brothers, and children developing cancer.

Importantly, we've recently discovered that tumors with BRCA mutations can be targeted with specific drugs, so their presence may also affect how we approach cancer treatment. These decisions affect people in very complicated ways. For instance, in a BRCA mutant patient who has a localized breast cancer, rather than undergoing a lumpectomy to remove her breast cancer, she may want to consider bilateral mastectomy and reconstruction so that she doesn't have to worry about developing a cancer in her other breast. There is also a higher risk of ovarian cancer in women who have a BRCA mutation, and we have a discussion with these women about the possibility of removing their ovaries and fallopian tubes before cancer develops. In women with a BRCA mutation, PARP inhibitors may be used to treat the cancer (see chapter 4).

It's important to remember that most breast cancers actually do not have a genetic basis. Scientists believe that about 75% of cancer is caused by the accumulation of random mutations, in other words, random chance. About 25% of cancers are caused by environmental factors, such as smoking, that accelerate the accumulation of mutations in cells or by inherited predisposition to cancer. People often think that if they have a history of breast cancer in their family, they must have inherited a gene that caused their cancer. In fact, only about 10% of breast cancers are thought to be hereditary. If your doctor thinks that genetic testing may be helpful for you, she may refer you to a cancer genetics professional who will talk to you about your family history. The discussion will include the pros and cons of genetic testing and whether to undertake it in your case. Genetic testing is performed on a sample of your blood or saliva. While this may seem simple, it's a test that requires informed consent. That means you need to have a discussion with your medical team and give consent to have this test done.

Who Should See a Genetics Counselor?

Your oncology team will consider various factors in determining whether you might benefit from meeting with a genetics counselor to discuss genetic testing. For example, your age at diagnosis is a consideration. If you are in your forties or younger at the time of diagnosis or if you are in your fifties and diagnosed with triple-negative breast cancer, your oncologist will usually recommend meeting with the genetics team. If you have a history of other cancers, your doctor may also discuss a genetics referral. Additionally, your oncologist will ask you about whether there is any cancer in your immediate and extended family. Depending on what types of cancer and in how many relatives are affected, your doctor may refer you to meet with a genetics counselor.

This consultation may take place at around the time of your diagnosis, especially if it might impact your treatment decisions. Certain genetic mutations predispose a woman to developing another breast cancer in the future. For some women, this information might affect the decision to undergo bilateral mastectomy over a lumpectomy for an early-stage cancer. For others, the genetic information won't change their immediate treatment plans, and these women may see the genetics team at a later point in treatment, if they wish. Your oncologist may also be able to discuss and order genetic testing, so not all patients need to see a genetic counselor to undergo testing.

Specific Genes and Syndromes

Most people have heard of the BRCA1 and BRCA2 mutations. Most women who test positive for a gene associated with an inherited breast cancer have one of these mutations. Yet, there are other genes that are associated with breast cancer. Examples of inherited genes that are associated with a higher risk of breast cancer include TP53, PALB2, PTEN, and CDH1. Other mutations are associated with a moderate increased risk of breast cancer. These include—but are not limited to—CHEK2,

ATM, and BRIP1. Some of these mutations are associated with cancers other than breast cancer. If your genetics report identifies one of these mutations, your genetics team and oncology team will talk to you about their recommendations, which may include adding on an annual breast MRI to routine annual mammograms.

What If My Results Are Negative?

If you have genetic testing and the results are negative, this means that a mutation was not found. However, a negative result needs some interpretation in the context of your family history. If your family members have a genetic mutation that is known to increase the risk of breast cancer, a negative test means that you did not inherit this mutation. This means that you do not have a known mutation that you could pass on to your children. We call this a true negative test. In other words, we think that your cancer is most likely due to random chance and that you don't have to worry about passing an inherited predisposition onto your kids.

If you come from a family with multiple cases of cancer and there is not a known genetic mutation in your family, a negative test is considered an uninformative negative. This means that with the data we have now, you do not have a mutation that is known to predispose to cancer. However, this does not guarantee that you do not have a genetic basis for your cancer, as there may still be an undiscovered genetic mutation.

Another important finding on genetic testing is something called a variant of uncertain significance (VUS). This means that a variation was found in a specific gene but it is unclear whether this might put you at a higher risk of cancer. This can be hard to understand and cope with, and it's important to talk to your team about these results. Sometimes a VUS gets reclassified as something benign, meaning that with more information scientists have figured out that the variation in your gene is not something that is thought to increase your risk of cancer. But sometimes a VUS gets reclassified as malignant, meaning it does result in an increased risk of cancer. If you have a VUS, it's important to follow up with a genetics counselor every two years or so.

CHAPTER SIX

How Am I Supposed to Cope Emotionally?

A diagnosis of breast cancer can affect every area of your life, and the busier and more active you were before your diagnosis, the more you can feel that your life has been derailed, and the more coping strategies you are going to need to get yourself back on track. Carla was in her late forties when she was diagnosed with metastatic triple-negative breast cancer. Before her diagnosis, she was in the middle of a master of fine arts program that she started after her two kids went off to college, and she was an avid hiker who spent most weekends in the woods of western Massachusetts with her dog. She had been hoping to earn her graduate degree and start teaching full time.

One day I (Vicki) asked her how she was doing with her daily life, and she said, "I can't believe how much has changed in three months. Everything has been taken over by treatments. I can't do any of the things I love to do. I don't know how to make any plans for the future."

This feeling is completely normal. What Carla needed, and what all newly diagnosed patients need, is a plan B, along with some strategies for coping with these overwhelming feelings. This starts with figuring out what's important to you and what you can do given your health status and energy level.

Carla thought about what was important to her. She knew that her energy was lower than normal and that she wanted to use the energy she did have for her boys, who frequently came home from college to see her. She decided to quit her MFA program, but she also wanted to do something that brought meaning to her life. She started volunteering in the office of the local animal shelter. She also had to figure out how to be out in the woods even if she didn't feel up to doing her usual five-mile hikes. Lastly, she had to find foods to eat other than the pastas she used to love because they just didn't appeal to her anymore.

Many people feel powerless in the first months after diagnosis. It's tempting to feel that your life has ended, but it hasn't. Your life has taken a turn that you hadn't envisioned, but you can adapt. You can learn how to live with cancer. You have the power to be engaged with what's happening and make your life the best it can be.

I wrote in chapter 1 about the positive health effects of palliative care. Research has long shown that cancer patients who get palliative care from the time of diagnosis are more likely to have an improved quality of life and better mental health outcomes. The question was why. What is the cause of these positive effects? The newest studies show that patients who receive palliative care cope differently than those who don't. In fact, coping is a big part of what we talk about in palliative care appointments. I talk to my patients about how they are feeling and give them some strategies for framing the big changes in their lives while also continuing to set goals for themselves. These are important skills.

Learning to cope effectively while living with a breast cancer diagnosis means having a safe place to talk about the ways in which the cancer has changed your life while finding ways to stay engaged in the world. Social workers can be very helpful with this. A palliative care clinician can help you strategize about how to set goals and manage fatigue and other symptoms so you can do more of what you want. In this chapter, I'll describe coping strategies that will make it easier to get through each day.

Why Me?

It is normal to look for something or someone to blame. You may be feeling that your health choices or lifestyle choices may have led you to this point. Patients often ask their doctors whether they did something to cause the cancer. The short answer is no. Although, technically, individuals can put themselves at an increased risk of getting cancer through certain behaviors, there is no direct line between a particular behavior and definitely getting cancer. Not everyone who smokes gets lung cancer, and some people get lung cancer even though they have never smoked. A big part of cancer is just random chance. Your cancer diagnosis is not a punishment for past behavior, nor is it a punishment for failing to get certain health screenings.

Ultimately, cancer is a biological process and mostly beyond your control. I stress this because I have had patients who insist that their impeccable health choices should have exempted them from cancer. People say to me, "I run five miles a day. I drink kale smoothies. I meditate.

I'm kind to animals. How can this be happening?" And I hear you. You may have been hoping that your terrific health choices would count for something. Secretly, you may have wanted them to transform themselves into a "get out of jail free" card for cancer. While it's normal for these thoughts to cross your mind from time to time, you don't want to cling to them. Over time, this belief that you ought to have a special health status will drain your energy. It's similar to the belief that some people have that they will be cured as long as they only think positive thoughts. Oncologists sometimes call this "the tyranny of optimism," because this belief becomes so exhausting for patients and their families and yet is so pervasive in the larger culture.

You can waste a lot of energy telling yourself that you deserve a certain outcome in treatment because you never smoked or never ate meat or never missed a workout. But, in reality, the best course of action now is to engage with a good treatment team and make a good plan to treat the cancer.

Coping Doesn't Mean Fighting

In the larger culture people often refer to coping with cancer as a battle and the illness as something that must be fought if it is ever going to be defeated. In some ways this is a comforting metaphor for any serious illness, because you can cast the illness as the villain and yourself as the hero who will fight at all costs. If you are supporting someone who has cancer, you may use this metaphor because it means that all of your sacrifices and hard work are part of this critical battle. But this metaphor has limitations, specifically because it stresses that dealing with cancer ultimately divides patients into winners and losers. If the treatments work well and the tumors shrink, it's great to feel like a winner. But what if the biology of the cancer doesn't allow for this? You are not a loser if your cancer advances.

Having worked with thousands of patients, I can tell you that the patients who cope best in this new world of cancer treatment are the ones who give up on the notion that they can push the cancer away by fighting it, being tough enough, or by enduring treatments and side effects stoically.

Also, breast cancer is unique in that it comes with an entire social movement attached to it. Breast cancer primarily affects women, and the pink ribbons, social awareness campaigns, online communities, and fundraising have all done enormous good. Many, many women feel connected to and empowered by this large, supportive network of patients and survivors. This social movement values self-education and optimism. It tells women that they are strong and that they matter. All of these are great messages.

My one concern is that many of my patients feel that they should be able to do everything they did before the diagnosis with the same grace, skill, and selflessness. They feel that they are expected to achieve at work and be supportive to their families at home no matter what they are going through physically and emotionally. I worry about this because the battle metaphor doesn't leave a lot of room for the actual coping techniques that will be most effective. I see many beautiful strong women who exhibit their strength by living well *with* their cancer, and for those who have metastatic cancer, by beginning to plan for a time when they are facing the end of their life.

Often the patients who cope most successfully come to feel that cancer is a kind of partner in their lives. That may sound strange, because of course you would never have chosen cancer as a partner or wished it on anyone else. But altering your metaphor from a battle to a partnership allows you to spend your energy working around the cancer and all of the changes it has brought to your life. You can try to enjoy what's going on in your life in spite of treatments. You may want to find ways to celebrate or treat yourself on the days when you feel most energetic. Later on, you may be surprised to find that cancer has altered your life in positive ways as well.

One of my patients with early-stage breast cancer, who I had been seeing for about eighteen months, confessed to me that she had never felt closer to her adult children as she had during treatment. Both of her children lived busy lives in other states and had the habit of coming home only briefly on major holidays. Since her diagnosis, they used their vacations and family leave to come home and stay with her for weeks at a time. She did perfectly ordinary things with them—baking, watching old home movies, going out to lunch—but for her these were treasured times, a chance to reconnect with her adult children in a new way, not only as a mother but as a person. "This would never have happened if I didn't have cancer," she told me. That is not to say that she liked having cancer. She didn't. But she was able to appreciate that it had brought new focus and urgency to her family relationships even though her cancer had a high likelihood of cure.

Symptom Management

The first step in effective coping is to make sure you can talk to your doctor about your symptoms and any side effects of the cancer treatment itself. It's going to be harder to make plans for doing things you love and finding ways to cope emotionally if you are undertreating any pain that you have or if your doctor doesn't know that you have neuropathy (numbness or pain in your hands and feet) or nausea or bowel troubles. I urge patients to keep a daily diary of symptoms and reactions to medications. Your oncologist is undoubtedly busy and probably focused on tests and scans and trying to make sure your anti-cancer therapies are working the way they should. Plan to bring a list of your top three symptom concerns to each visit and ask how your medical team can help you with them.

Using Multiple Strategies

Like Carla, many people use physical activity as a way to stay fit and also as a way to discharge stress. You may have enjoyed running or swimming or lifting weights as a way to calm down and feel centered before your cancer diagnosis. You can certainly modify your workouts to do them for as long as possible. I've worked with patients who loved yoga, and together we modified poses for them to do on those days when they were dealing with fatigue or pain. There will likely be times during your treatment when your favorite fitness activities are difficult or no longer possible. Exceptionally driven people sometimes feel defeated when they can't exercise. I urge patients to find other coping strategies to turn to on those days when their usual exercise regimen is not an option.

Coping Strategies

Your ability to cope is like the weather in that it's different every day. Some days you may feel that you aren't coping particularly well, but don't get down on yourself. Some days are just going to suck. But having a bad day doesn't mean that you are getting worse or that you are doomed to have more bad days. Be kind to yourself on those days when you may be particularly cranky or out of it. Tomorrow you will probably feel different, and you can start again.

These are the strategies my patients often use successfully to cope with cancer and to live full lives in spite of it: distraction, optimism, gratitude, joy, meditation and prayer, humor, flow, intellectualizing, and problem solving. You may already use two or three of the following activities to help with stress. Many people have just one favorite coping strategy. But I encourage you to try several and see what works for you. It is often good to have multiple strategies.

Distraction

This is perhaps the easiest coping technique, made even easier by smartphone games, Internet surfing, and binge-watching favorite TV shows. Yes, there are times when you can—and should—distract yourself from thoughts about cancer or your symptoms and side effects. You may need distraction when waiting for test results or scans seems especially difficult or on those days when you feel more fatigued. One of my patients loves to watch the "bird cam" at Cornell Labs and also one of the many panda cams at various zoos because watching animals is relaxing for her. When she can't sleep, she listens to podcasts so she can learn new things, and when she is anxious, she plays games on her smartphone. "They all tell me I'm obsessed," she says about reactions from her friends and family. But it's a healthy obsession because it helps her cope. Other people spend the afternoon watching romantic comedies or classic hockey games. The point is to pass the time enjoyably while giving yourself a break.

Optimism

You can harness the power of optimism by creating some event to look forward to. Think of something that will give you pleasure, and make time to do it in the near future. This might be attending a child or grandchild's recital, going shopping, calling a friend you haven't talked to in a while to set up a coffee date, or looking forward to watching a sporting event. You can make small plans, such as taking a day off from work to go to a matinee, or you can make big plans, such as taking a dream trip. One patient told herself that if she got through a difficult surgery, she would plan her dream trip to Paris. She later said, "As soon as I got home from the hospital, I was on the Internet pricing flights and looking into hotel rooms." The ability to anticipate something and look forward to it—even if it's many months away—can change your whole outlook on life in general. Yes, there is uncertainty. Thankfully, there are a lot of excellent travel insurance options to hedge your bets.

Gratitude

In the field of positive psychology, the concept of gratitude is getting a lot of attention. Several experiments have shown that people who can write down three things for which they are grateful, and do this every day, have a better outlook on life and even have healthier relationships and life habits. Can you find and name three things for which you are grateful? You might be grateful for the companionship of a pet, a beautiful tree in your backyard, a partner who is supportive, getting your favorite infusion nurse, or a coworker's sense of humor. On some days, finding something specific to name may seem difficult, but you will get better at it with practice. Ultimately, you may develop a skill that we call Velcro versus Teflon. The good things in your life will stick to you like Velcro, because you concentrate on them, while the bad things you will notice and deal with before letting them slide off of you like Teflon.

Joy

Take as many opportunities as you can to stay in the moment and enjoy simple things: a sunset, a well-played game of baseball, a good joke, a hug, a connection with a friend, nature in any form. This is something people rarely take the time to do, to really appreciate experiences as they are happening. One of my patients who lives on Cape Cod told me that she loves using her outdoor shower and now uses it all the time because it feels so good to be outside. This is using joy as a coping strategy— doing something that feels good and enjoying every minute of it. Another patient told me that putting up Christmas decorations had always seemed like a chore, the first of so many to get through in an endless to-do list every December, but this year she decided that she would slow down and make hanging ornaments into an event. She also decided to go through the entire season doing only what she wanted to do, only what she knew she would enjoy.

Meditation and Prayer

Some of my patients had been meditating for many years before their cancer diagnoses, while others try it for the first time after a diagnosis or well into their treatment regimens as a way of escaping the loop of worrying thoughts. People with a strong connection to a religious tradition may find prayer helpful on those days when coping seems especially difficult. Regardless of your spiritual tradition or beliefs, time for reflection is an important way to stay centered. There are many phone apps that offer a variety of guided mediations that can be a helpful way to start a medication practice.

Humor

Tanya is a patient of mine who was quite happy with the reconstructive surgery she had after her mastectomy. During an appointment with her husband and her children she said, "I had been thinking about a little lift, but who knew I would get this fabulous entire boob job?" Her husband chimed in without missing a beat and said to her, "Seriously, if you wanted the whole megillah, we could have talked about it. You didn't have to go ahead and get cancer just to get the top of the line deal here." Tanya and her husband burst out laughing, while their children looked at each other nervously.

Many people have a great sense of humor and use laughter as a primary coping mechanism, and yet patients still sometimes ask whether it's okay to make jokes about having cancer. Of course it is! You have to endure a lot of craziness with cancer, and it's okay to laugh when you can and to be snarky, even edgy. No one will be offended—least of all your oncologist or your palliative care clinician. They've heard it all.

Flow

This is another concept from the field of positive psychology, and it refers to any activity that causes you to feel immersed in energized focus, involvement, and enjoyment of the process. It's different from distraction because you are doing something active and creative that is challenging without being overwhelmingly difficult. You may also think of this as being "in the zone," and some people find this feeling through work or through such creative activities as knitting, writing, or playing an instrument.

One of my patients loves painting, and she belongs to a painting club. Every two weeks, club members meet in a set location, either at the local high school or rec center, and paint together. She loves it because she can lose herself in the painting and not think of anything else. She loves the smell of the paints and the camaraderie of the fellow painters, and even though she sometimes finds it difficult to get out of the house, she is always grateful to go to these club meetings. The idea is to find an activity that will challenge you creatively or intellectually enough to allow you to get outside yourself and to continue to grow.

Intellectualization

This is a technique you can use when you want to treat cancer the way you treat other problems, as intellectual puzzles. You may want to spend a lot of time researching all of the chemical compounds in your chemotherapy drugs and learn all about the mechanisms of how they act on cancer cells. You may want to come up with graphs and charts for the side effects of treatments. You may want to research religious and spiritual texts and think about the meaning of life. These are great coping strategies because they help you deal with the fact of cancer without having to think about the emotional component of your diagnosis and treatment all the time.

Problem Solving

This is a great technique on those days when you want to feel like you've accomplished something. This may mean researching alternative therapies with the plan of discussing them with your doctor. You may decide to make a financial plan to help take care of your family. You may be focused on fixing up the house, thinking, "I'm finally going to repair that cabinet door," or "Today is the day I'm going to clean out those files." Finding practical tasks to do and problems to solve will give you a sense of control at a time when so much may seem to be out of your control.

Building a Community

A cancer diagnosis can be an incredibly isolating experience. Even your closest friends and family may not understand what you are going through. Participating in a support group can be a way to share this experience with others who deeply understand what it's like to go through treatment and to live with the possibility of recurrence. Online breast cancer communities and blogs can offer advice about navigating the cancer experience as well as emotional support.

You can also join a larger community of women living with breast cancer and those who care about them. The pink ribbon signifies this solidarity and community. It is a visible way to show support for those in treatment. Many organizations support breast cancer awareness programs, fundraisers, research, and support groups. It is hard to overstate how important it is have others who understand the physical and identity issues and the uncertainty that accompany a diagnosis of breast cancer.

Talking and Thinking About Difficult Topics

Part of coping is finding a way to think about and talk about difficult topics. The most important of these is the question of what you plan to do if your cancer recurs or if the treatments don't work as well as you hope. Some people are comfortable with making plans for a future in which the illness may be even more prominent in their lives, while other patients tell me that they don't want to talk about or even think about any negative possibilities. They want to focus on the idea of being cured or of dealing with the cancer as a chronic illness. One patient said to me, "I don't want to think about anything other than making the cancer go away, because if I sit around worrying about dying, I'm just inviting the cancer to get worse." I had to respectfully disagree with her on several points.

First, I know that talking about a possibility doesn't make it come true. Cancer cells are driven by their own biology and not by your thoughts or anyone else's. I also know that her stated concern about wanting to think only positive thoughts was masking several other concerns that are normal and realistic. If you are dealing with a cancer diagnosis, you may be afraid that if you thoroughly consider all of the possible outcomes, you might become overwhelmed and depressed and unable to think about anything else or enjoy your life. Some people say to me, "I'm afraid that if I start crying, I may never stop." These are real concerns.

I also know that refusing to talk about your fears and about possible outcomes doesn't work very well. Think about it. It would be crazy to never have any fears or negative thoughts. So, in reality, you are not keeping the negative thoughts away; you're just sealing them off in a pressure cooker that is sure to explode later. People who try to stay stoic during the day often find that they lie awake at night or that they develop panic attacks or struggle more with fatigue. Rather than avoiding negative thoughts, you will want to find a safe way to talk about difficult topics, including your prognosis (the likely course and outcome of your disease) and what plans you may need to make if your cancer progresses. By talking about these issues and giving voice to your fears, you are taking away their power over you. It may actually be easier to get back to your life after discharging your fears, if you do it in a safe way.

Opening the Box

With my patients, I often use the metaphor of the box. Everything they don't want to have to talk about or think about goes in the box. So I ask, "Do you want to talk about your prognosis?" If the answer is no, this conversation goes in the box. "Do you want to talk about what might happen if your cancer grows through this treatment?" No? It goes in the box. We don't have to open the box until you are ready, but at some point we may have to open the box, even if it's just for a few minutes. Most patients love this idea because it gives them control over when they feel ready to talk about what may be bothering them.

I have a patient with metastatic breast cancer, and she has been in treatment for almost three years. She's an intense, hard-driven person who truly believes that you can get a good outcome in anything if you work hard enough. She was initially resistant to talking about the possibility of any negative outcomes, but lately she has been wanting to open the box and have these conversations about what might happen if she can't get into a clinical trial as she hopes or what might happen if her scans show additional metastases. Considering all possibilities gives her the power to decide whether to get a particular cancer treatment. She can talk about how to encourage her husband to engage support services if her health gets worse. And then, when we close the box, she can go right back to talking about how she believes the right clinical trial is going to open up for her, even though she knows it's a long shot. Opening the box allows her to talk realistically about what might happen, while staying hopeful about everything else.

You can use this box idea with your doctor; you can even use it with your family. The point is to allow you and your family to stay hopeful while making room to talk about and plan for the challenges you might have to deal with, even if you don't want them to happen.

Coping with Other People

Patients sometimes tell me that the hardest challenge (emotionally) to deal with in the world of cancer is the feeling that their friends and loved ones don't know what to say and maybe even make themselves scarce for weeks or months at a time. In fact, your diagnosis may be so worrisome for other people that they either avoid the topic altogether or ask annoying and prying questions about what you are going through. In fact, there is a new line of greeting cards by Emily McDowell that captures some of this awkwardness. The message on one card reads, "I'm really sorry I haven't been in touch. I didn't know what to say." Another one says, "I promise never to try to sell you on some random treatment I read on the Internet."

It's normal to feel a little isolated at the start of treatment while you are sorting out which of your friends and family members are going to actively support you at this time and which are going to fade into the outer circle. For some people, talking about anything that raises the idea of mortality is too much; some would rather say and do nothing than say the wrong thing while trying to help out. Figure out who you can rely on the most and how to manage the flow of information to extended family and friends.

The Inner and Outer Orbits

It's normal to wonder how you can talk to your friends about what's going on in your life and how to ask for the support you truly need. People often tell me that they need their friends and close family so much but don't want to overburden them. Feeling like a burden is common. What I suggest is thinking of friends and loved ones in terms of one inner circle and several outer circles.

The friends who are in your innermost orbit are the friends you know and trust the most. These are the people (and there may be just one or two) who can come to your house unannounced, ignore any clutter or mess, and when you offer to make them coffee, cheerfully make it themselves because they already know their way around your kitchen. These are the people you will rely on the most, for errands, for companionship, and for commiseration. They are the ones who will never think of you as a burden. They may be terribly sad about the turn of events, but they are also the ones who can see you at your worst and roll with it. Cherish them.

Your other close friends and family—the outer orbits—may need a little help with this cancer thing, even if they love you very much. You may not feel as comfortable asking for help, and they may be less available to give it. You may have to rehearse what to say when they lower their voices and say, "How are you doing?" while looking worried. It's okay. You can come up with a pat answer to have ready, and the moment will pass. People need guidance and direction because they don't know how to say or do helpful things. The point is to speak up when you are uncomfortable. I have one patient who gets angry when family members talk about her as though she is not in the room. One of them will say, "Who is going to take Mary to the store?" And she's thinking, "I'm Mary. I'm right here. Talk to me!" She's brilliant but feels that sometimes people treat her as though she is helpless. But she's getting better at standing up for herself.

Another one of my patients was at a holiday dinner when a distant cousin turned to her and said, "Did you lose your hair everywhere?" It was an awkward moment to be sure, but at least she has a funny story to tell. The very subject of cancer is frightening to some people who have no experience with it, and they sometimes say things they immediately regret. Or maybe they regret it the next day but are too embarrassed to reach out with an apology.

Many patients learn to treat all of this with great humor. I have one patient who actually made what she called Cancer Cards. They were real cards with the word "cancer" printed on them. And when she wanted to get her way with a quarrelsome family member, she would whip out one of the cards and say, "I'm playing the cancer card." She literally trumped other people's views. Once I think she had one of the cards with her at an amusement park, and instead of waiting in the long line with her grandchild, she went to the front of the line and presented the card to the attendant, and said, "Excuse me, I have cancer." This was a little bit later in her illness, when she was aware of time running short. The attendant took the card, and no one objected. Sometimes it's okay to play the cancer card.

Asking for Help

Some people find it difficult to ask anyone, even close friends and family, to help them get along day to day because they don't want to feel like a burden. A patient of mine, Jessica, was in her early thirties and a successful entrepreneur when she was diagnosed with breast cancer. She elected to have a double mastectomy. Initially after the surgery, she was deeply conflicted about having anyone help her. She believed that she needed to maintain her independence and do everything for herself. She thought it would help her family feel more confident about how she was coping if she told them she didn't need any help after surgery. In truth, they just became more worried. They called constantly asking whether she needed any help and offering to shop and cook for her. Her parents were beside themselves imagining that she was feeling awful in her apartment by herself.

After several tense exchanges with her family, Jessica realized she needed a different approach. She made a list of everything that would make her life easier if someone could help, including laundry, grocery shopping, and being with her to get back and forth to the clinic when she started chemotherapy. She told me she realized that friends and family couldn't go through the cancer treatment but she could let them be connected with her by letting them help. She told me, "The best way I can love them is by letting them help me. It just took me a while to figure that one out."

Extended Family and Community

Those closest to you will be in contact with you every day and may even come to appointments with you. But what about everybody else? If you have a large extended family or a large social network, you may want to have someone send a group email with some basic facts about your diagnosis and what kind of help would be appreciated. I know of one rabbi who did this for his wife. He sent out a group email to the members of his temple to inform them of her breast cancer diagnosis. What was great about this letter is that it reassured his congregation that his wife was getting excellent care and didn't have any immediate needs. It was also clear about what the couple did and didn't want in terms of communication. It stated that while they welcomed good thoughts and prayers, they didn't want to receive phone calls or emails in the near term. The couple felt an obligation to be honest with members, but they also knew that the last thing they needed was an endlessly ringing phone so that people could say some version of "I'm sorry." If you are going to send out a group email, it's important to state what you do and don't want from the people receiving it.

The rabbi's letter also directed recipients to a website where a temple member was coordinating efforts to help the couple. There are several websites that do this. One of them is called Care Calendar, and another is called Lotsa Helping Hands. These websites become a clearinghouse for coordinating all kinds of help, including prepared meals, visits from friends, dog walking, or rides to medical appointments. These kinds of websites give people concrete ways to offer help, which makes them feel so much better than offering the vague, "Let me know if I can do anything."

Some people start a blog to keep everyone informed of what they are going through and what they are thinking along the way. What's great about this is that you can include as much or as little information as you like. Even if you don't use a website or blog, you can assign someone to serve as the communications czar, the person who will get medical updates to extended family and who will field questions people may not be comfortable asking you directly. This person can also set up a schedule for others who want to help with visits or giving the kids rides to school. This can make a big difference for you and give people an opportunity to support you in ways that you truly need.

Coping after Treatment

People who are treated for early-stage breast cancer sometimes struggle with returning to their normal lives after completing such intensive treatments as surgery, chemotherapy, and radiation therapy. Many patients feel both excitement and anxiety as they complete breast cancer treatment. Sometimes women are so glad to be done with treatment and don't look back; other times patients really struggle with returning to their normal day-to-day lives. Some find the routine of lab draws, visits with a team they have come to trust, and seeing their infusion nurse a comforting routine that is hard to let go of. Others find it disconcerting to enter back into their lives where their friends, family, and colleagues seem unchanged, while they have been affected deeply by the experience of cancer.

One such story comes from Jenn, who met with Lakshmi for her first visit after completing a vigorous regimen of chemotherapy for early-stage HER2-positive breast cancer. Lakshmi said she thought she would feel happier to be done. Instead, she said that she was struggling with being back at work. While her colleagues were incredibly supportive, Lakshmi said it was hard to keep hearing, "You look great!" Everyone seemed to expect her to be the same Lakshmi she was before the cancer diagnosis, but the experience had left her shaken. She was also feeling anxious about recurrence and not seeing her medical team as frequently as she had been during her chemotherapy treatments.

Jenn sometimes describes this stage of posttreatment as "re-entry." She makes the analogy of a spacecraft returning to Earth's atmosphere. Talk to your oncology team about how you are feeling so that they can provide support and guidance. Many patients find it reassuring to know that others experience similar challenges.

CHAPTER SEVEN

How Do I Cope with Changes in My Body?

Jenn, Dave, and I are often told that the physical changes brought about by breast cancer treatment are the most challenging to deal with. Patients say, "My body is so different. I don't recognize myself anymore." Breast cancer treatment can bring noticeable weight changes or hair loss or surgery that alters your body. It's tough to look at yourself in the bathroom mirror and see scars or changes in your breasts, or an arm swollen from lymphedema, or to walk differently because of neuropathy. A big part of living well with cancer is figuring out who you are in this new body and how you relate to others, even though you may be wondering whether they look at you differently and whether they see you as a cancer patient rather than a person.

It's hard to know which changes are going to be the most difficult for you. I saw a woman at the clinic recently who had been living with breast cancer for more than five years. Julie had gone through a mastectomy and several cycles of chemotherapy in which she had lost a significant amount of weight. And yet she prided herself on not letting the diagnosis define her. She continued to work nearly full time, and she still went to the gym several times per week. Now, for the first time, she was losing her hair as a result of treatment. Julie told me how strange it was to look at herself in the mirror with her new wig. "I feel like a cancer patient now," Julie said to me. "I haven't until this point." For her, the idea that acquaintances and strangers would look at her differently was the hardest part. She worried that wearing a wig was like wearing a sign that says, "I have cancer." And she worried that people would want her to talk about her diagnosis even when she didn't feel like talking about it.

In this chapter, I'll describe some ways to cope with these physical changes that can be temporary, such as hair loss, or that are permanent, such as changes to your breasts. And I'll talk about changes in intimate relationships and sexual function and how to cope with those.

Hair Loss

Losing hair is hard for almost everyone but especially for women, because women live with a cultural expectation of having not just hair but a hairstyle. Women often tell me that this is the side effect they fear most, and then they minimize this worry by adding, "I know it should be the least of my concerns." But hair loss doesn't have to be the least of your concerns. It's normal to feel a personal sense of loss when the reflection in the mirror is different than what we are used to seeing. There are many reasons why hair loss or thinning can be emotionally difficult to anticipate and experience.

I advise people to ask their oncology teams about the likelihood that any regimen will result in hair loss and when it might occur. If you are being treated with chemotherapy for an early-stage breast cancer, hair loss is an expected side effect of the chemotherapy treatment. Your doctor may speak with you about the option of cold caps, which are more effective with certain chemotherapy regimens as compared to others (chapter 4). If you are being treated with chemotherapy for advanced breast cancer, talk to your doctor about the impact of treatment on hair loss and thinning since not all regimens cause this side effect.

Oncologists and oncology nurses know how different regimens often affect patients. Still, they may not always be accurate, as everyone reacts differently. Julie had told me that her oncologist estimated that just 5% of people lose their hair on her regimen, and she turned out to be in that minority. So she was happy that she had gone to a wig store to get a high-quality wig made before she lost her hair. The fitter was able to see how she wore her hair while she had it and crafted a wig that was in keeping with that style. Wigs can be expensive, depending on the type that you choose, and many insurers don't cover this cost. Also, wigs made of 100% human hair often need more upkeep than those made of other materials. Some people ultimately don't like wearing a wig and opt for scarves or hats instead. Julie's concerns about wearing a wig eased when she realized that some coworkers didn't notice it, and those who may have noticed knew better than to comment.

There is a lot of advice online about how to manage the actual hair loss as it's happening. Sometimes hair loss is gradual and sometimes rapid, and you may see advice to keep your hair cropped close or to shave your head as the thinning progresses to keep from dealing with hair coming out in clumps. After you experience hair loss, you may notice that you get cold more easily and that the skin on your scalp is more sensitive and more vulnerable to sunburn.

If you are being treated with chemotherapy for early-stage breast cancer, your hair will grow back when the treatment regimen ends. If you are on treatments for advanced cancer that cause hair thinning or loss, your hair might start to grow back if you switch to a new treatment that does not impact the hair. Hair should start to regrow about three weeks after your last treatment. Interestingly enough, your hair may even grow back with a different texture or color than it was previously. It's not unusual for hair to grow back curly in a person who has had straight hair her whole life.

Neuropathy

Some patients experience pronounced neuropathy during chemotherapy treatments for early- or late-stage breast cancer. They may have numbness, tingling, or pain in their hands or feet. These symptoms can interfere with writing and typing or fastening buttons. Some people have decreased sensation in their feet, affecting the way they walk. They may have to step carefully. I've had patients say that their grandkids ask them why they suddenly seem so frail. And they feel frail, as though their bodies don't work as well as they should. Avid golfers have trouble setting up shots or walking through a golf course because they have lost a strong sense of balance.

One of my patients loved sailing, and she also experienced very mild balance issues from chemotherapy-induced neuropathy. She had no issues while walking, but she noted mild symptoms while at sea. She decided to hold off on sailing in races for several months, and as her neuropathy improved and eventually resolved, she was able to get back to sailing competitively. Dave usually tells patients that it can take months for neuropathy to heal, and sometimes you won't feel normal again for up to a year. But when you stop using the chemotherapy regimen that is causing the nerve problems, most neuropathies will resolve over time. Others get better but never completely go away.

If you are being treated with a chemotherapy that is known to cause neuropathy, your doctors will be asking you about any numbness, tingling, burning, or pain in your hands or feet. Be sure to let your team know if your symptoms are getting worse over time and not resolving between your treatments. If the neuropathy is getting worse, your doctor may talk to you about holding treatment for a week or reducing the dose. People often worry about delaying chemotherapy or getting a lower dose, and your doctor will help you understand the benefits and the risks for you.

When Jenn was meeting with Svetlana, she was being treated with her last cycle of paclitaxel for an early-stage breast cancer. She had been doing well on therapy, noticing only some mild pins and needles in her fingertips. These sensations lasted just a few days after each of her first two paclitaxel treatments. After her third paclitaxel treatment, she said that the pins and needles became more like electric shocks in her feet that weren't going away. She was a bartender and had to take time off after her most recent treatment because it was too painful to be on her feet for an entire shift. The pain was also making it hard to sleep at night. This is the kind of disruptive side effect that we want to minimize. Jenn suggested holding treatment for one week and reducing that final dose by 20%, and Svetlana was initially nervous about going off schedule. Jenn explained that a delay was not likely to derail her progress. Instead, it would give her symptoms a chance to resolve. When she returned the following week pain free, she was relieved that she felt so much better. Ultimately, her last cycle of chemotherapy went well.

Your oncologist may also talk to you about the option of using medication to help ease the symptoms of neuropathy. Gabapentin and duloxetine are two commonly prescribed medications that may help treat the symptoms of numbness, tingling, and discomfort in the fingers and toes. These may be prescribed during chemotherapy or even after you have completed treatment.

Lymphedema

As mentioned in chapter 3, you may experience swelling in your arm from lymphedema. This can happen if you have had surgery to remove lymph nodes in your armpit. The risk of lymphedema increases with the number of lymph nodes removed. You are also at a higher risk if you've had radiation treatments. Lymphedema can also occur in a patient with metastatic breast cancer who has not had any lymphatic surgery, if tumors develop in the lymph nodes or block drainage of the lymph vessels.

Lymphedema may impact your quality of life in several ways. The arm can become swollen and heavy and the skin can become tight. You may experience numbness or tingling in the arm or a sense that it is less flexible. You may be prescribed a glove or sleeve, called a compression sleeve, to help decrease the swelling. For some, swelling and use of a compression sleeve are a constant reminder of a breast cancer diagnosis.

If you experience lymphedema, your oncology team can refer you to a physical therapist who can help with manually decompressing your arm with massage to drain the lymph nodes. He or she may also recommend certain compression garments. If the swelling is more severe, the physical therapist may recommend devices that use a sleeve or stocking that can be intermittently inflated over the affected arm, in addition to the manual decompression and sleeves. It's important to let your doctor know if you've detected any changes to your arm. In some cases, your doctor may advise checking for a blood clot in your arm or making sure that cancer has not returned.

There are also some surgical procedures that may help treat lymphedema. However, there are no robust studies showing that these surgeries are effective, and they are not widely available. One surgery uses liposuction of the affected arm followed by bandaging and constant compression. Another involves transferring healthy lymph nodes from one part of the body to the armpit region. A third entails bridging the lymphatic vessels to the veins in the armpit. These surgeries generally do not cure lymphedema, and the mainstay treatments are physical therapy and compression.

Early Menopause

Some breast cancer therapies may cause your body to enter menopause. If you are being treated with chemotherapy, your body many either temporarily or permanently enter into menopause. If you are being treated with drugs to suppress the ovaries or if you have had your ovaries removed, this will trigger a state of menopause as well. The experience of menopause varies greatly for women, with some experiencing no bothersome symptoms to others whose quality of life is impacted by hot flashes, vaginal dryness, and changes in libido, which is discussed toward the end of this chapter. These symptoms can be hard to handle on top of all the other things you are going through as you cope with the diagnosis and your treatments. We will address some of them and how to cope in chapter 8 since many of the symptoms of menopause are similar to those side effects experienced from hormonal therapies.

Getting Used to a New Body

Jenn's patients with early-stage cancer have gone through lumpectomies and mastectomies. Others with metastatic cancer did not have breast surgery and have a tumor within the breast that they can feel. Some of my patients with advanced cancer have a catheter in their lung or abdomen to drain fluid. In some cases, they take steroids or other medication that causes facial swelling, or they have bowel changes that mean they have to be near a bathroom much of the time. All of these changes make patients feel that they have exchanged their familiar body for something else, and it takes time to get used to this new body. There is a loss related to these changes, and it's absolutely normal to grieve these losses.

It's also important to figure out who you are in this new body and make strategies for how to live with these changes. This may mean asking questions about physical changes even before you have significant surgeries. Many of Jenn's patients debate between a lumpectomy or a mastectomy; others consider undergoing a double mastectomy (having both breasts removed). Women who choose mastectomy will also make the decision about whether to undergo breast reconstruction. Some women decide they don't want reconstruction and may consider whether they'd like to use a breast prosthesis, which may be made of foam or silicone and can sit within a bra to give the shape of a breast. Jenn encourages her patients to speak with the surgeon regarding what to expect in terms of how this might feel and what cosmetic results they might expect.

Even if you have done your research and had the opportunity to speak with your breast surgery team, though, it can be hard to know how you will feel after you've had your surgery. Many patients are pleasantly surprised after their surgery and are really pleased with the cosmetic results. Others struggle with looking or feeling different for various reasons. They may react to the new asymmetry of their breasts or the lack of sensation. Others admit to feeling less like a woman even if they are satisfied with how they look from the outside. It's normal to feel a range of emotions that might occur right after surgery or over time.

Some people put energy into looking as normal as possible because that gives them more confidence as they continue to work and socialize. One of my patients, Eva, worked in a hospital, and she said it was her goal to look as close to normal as possible. She wanted to provide some distance between herself and the cancer, especially at work, where she didn't want to have to answer questions about it. She had a wig styled to look exactly like her hair, and it did look exactly like her hair. Each time I walked into the room prior to her chemotherapy treatments, I had to do a double take because her hair looked so real.

For other patients, embracing their new normal is empowering to them, and I have had patients go completely bald and others who have bought wigs of different colors and styles. I'll never forget one of my young patients, Lisette, who brought in pictures of her modeling the five wigs she had purchased, two of which were in bright neon colors. Just like Eva and Lisette, you will figure out what works best for you as your body changes. Some women want to feel and look sexy because that's important to them, but this isn't a priority for everyone.

Many people feel alone at first in these changes because they have never known anyone who had to deal with these issues. But you aren't alone. There are lots of people going through the same challenges; many of them have written blogs about the experience or have created websites that detail great coping strategies. Some have even designed products to help others like themselves. By reading some of these accounts, you may find that these physical changes don't need to define you. They are simply part of the new you.

These body changes also may be unsettling for your partner. Remember that your partner may be grieving the loss of changes in your body and may need a little time to adjust. One of Jenn's patients, Zoe, had a mastectomy for an early-stage breast cancer with a plan to eventually undergo a breast reconstruction. She said that her wife was initially eager for her to have the reconstruction, and Zoe was as well, because she wanted to look like her old self. Over time, they both became more accustomed to her new body. Ultimately, Zoe decided that she did not want to pursue a breast reconstruction, and she said her wife was fully supportive of her decision.

Changes in Sexuality

My patients are sometimes reluctant to talk about how their cancer affects intimacy with their partners. People may have strong feelings about their new bodies that make it difficult to feel attractive or sexy. One of my patients who had a double mastectomy told me that it took her several months after her physical recovery before she felt like having sex again. "My husband told me that I was beautiful, and I believed him," she said. "And he told me that he didn't marry me for my breasts. I knew he was okay with it. I just needed some time to feel beautiful again in this new body, but it happened."

Cancer treatment can also change sexual function. It can affect sexual organs, functioning, and drive. Such treatments as chemotherapy and ovarian suppression can put you into menopause, and hormonal therapies can cause vaginal dryness or changes in libido. Sometimes factors related to the illness, like pain or fatigue, make actually having sex too tough. You don't have to assume that intercourse will be difficult forever, but it may be difficult right now. And I also remind people that sexual intercourse is just one way to be intimate with your partner.

Intimacy and Sex

Some couples feel that they ought to be having sex, even when intercourse has become tricky because of cancer treatment or when the libido is lower or even nil. Sometimes a woman with cancer feels a sense of obligation to her partner, and in some cases people think that having sex will make them feel more like themselves. Partners sometimes also want to initiate sex because they want to reaffirm the intimacy that they feel or because they want their partner to feel more whole and to feel loved and appreciated. Couples need to talk about these issues and see whether each person wants the same things. It's easy for couples to make assumptions about what the other person wants or needs emotionally and physically.

Cancer and treatment can affect your ability to have sex in the way you have before. Your doctor may not raise the issue of sexuality and sexual function, but continuing to be intimate with your partner is a meaningful part of living fully with cancer. Raising these issues with your medical team is part of advocating for yourself and your needs. Many large cancer centers have sexual health clinics and specialists who can help patients deal with the ways in which cancer has affected their sexuality.

I like to remind couples that intimacy isn't the same thing as having intercourse. They know this already, but it's good for people who have been coupled for a long time to remember that intimacy comes from all kinds of touching. Intercourse can give way to caressing, holding, hugging, and kissing. Holding your partner's hand is not the same as holding the hand of your child or your friend. You can maintain tremendous intimacy with your partner, even if you can't have sex in the way that you have in the past. The idea of intimacy can change and become much more emotional.

Sexual health specialists will also say that intimacy is sometimes a loaded word. It sounds like serious work, and in reality sex is a form of play. You can and should playfully explore the body that you have now, focusing on sensations. What feels good? Erogenous zones can change after cancer treatment, but they are still there. If intercourse is stressful, you can always step back to what else feels good.

Logistics of Intercourse

Many patients and their partners feel daunted by the logistics of sex. They have so many questions: Is it safe? Can my partner get exposed to the chemotherapy? Is there risk of infection? What if I get pregnant? What if it hurts? Let's address a few of these questions.

Is it safe? While the risk of passing chemotherapy to a partner is probably very small and largely unknown, some doctors will tell you to use a condom during the first two weeks after an infusion; others might say a condom is only necessary for the first 72 hours after an infusion.

Risk of infection. There are times after chemotherapy when you are at higher risk of developing an infection, and your team may advise against sexual intercourse during this time, usually seven to ten days after an infusion, when your white count is at its lowest point. Also, if your oncology team is worried about your risk of infection because you have a low white blood cell count, you will want to use condoms to minimize your exposure to sexually transmitted diseases.

Risk of pregnancy. Getting pregnant on most breast cancer treatments would not be safe. If you are not yet in menopause, talk to your doctor about what she recommends for contraception.

Pain management. If you have advanced breast cancer and cancer-related pain has been an issue, you will want to use proactive pain management. Some partners also worry that they will hurt the patient during sex. Work with your team to make sure your pain is well controlled. You may also need to premedicate with a breakthrough pain medication (see chapter 11) one hour before sex to ensure more comfort. I also remind people to think about different positions and ways of pleasuring yourself and your partner if intercourse is too painful. Sometimes side positions are easier and require less energy. But you might also consider alternative forms of sexual intimacy to penetration.

Fatigue. This is another common barrier to having sex and may require some planning to work around it because there aren't many treatments for fatigue. Most people with cancer-related fatigue do say there is a time of day when they feel most energetic. That would be a time to think about initiating sex. I also remind patients that fatigue gets worse when you have other symptoms that aren't controlled, so work with your medical team to treat them.

Vaginal dryness. If you are postmenopausal or have been made menopausal by chemotherapy or drugs that suppress the ovaries (e.g., leuprolide), you might experience vaginal symptoms such as dryness and pain with intercourse. Aromatase inhibitors may also contribute to this dryness (see chapter 8). We usually first recommend trying over-the-counter vaginal moisturizers and vaginal lubricants. Some women may also benefit from topical estrogens applied within the vagina.

For many, sexuality is an important quality of life issue. Your medical team may not bring this up, and I encourage you or your loved ones to discuss any concerns you might have with your team. The bottom line is that you should feel free to be open about all sexual issues with your treatment team. Some hospitals and practices have started dedicated sexual dysfunction clinics or have physicians who are known for their expertise in this area. Most oncologists can handle the basic questions and issues, but a dedicated specialist is often needed to answer more complex questions and issues. So ask your treatment team where you can get help for any sexual dysfunction.

Managing Symptoms and Side Effects

CHAPTER EIGHT

Managing the Side Effects of Hormonal Therapy

Hormonal therapies, also known as endocrine therapies, are some of the most commonly used drugs to treat breast cancer (see chapter 4). Specifically, they are used to treat women with breast cancers that have the estrogen or progesterone receptor, although some tumors have both receptors. Tumors that have these receptors are said to be estrogen receptor–positive and/or progesterone receptor–positive. Some people use the term *hormone receptor–positive* more generally. Having this receptor means that estrogen can stimulate a tumor cell to grow and replicate. Hormonal therapies block estrogen from binding to cell receptors, or prevent the body from creating estrogen. This blocks tumor cells from growing and replicating.

The most common hormonal therapies are tamoxifen, which can be used in women who are premenopausal or postmenopausal, and the aromatase inhibitors (aromatase being an enzyme that helps the body synthesize estrogen from fat cells), which are used in women who are postmenopausal. There are three aromatase inhibitors: anastrozole, letrozole, and exemestane. Tamoxifen and the aromatase inhibitors are all oral medications. Fulvestrant, on the other hand, is a medication that is given in the muscle (usually in the buttocks) and binds to the estrogen receptor, thus making the receptor unable to bind to estrogen.

Doctors may also use shots to suppress ovarian function and cause menopause in someone who has not yet gone through a natural menopause. Leuprolide (Lupron) and goserelin (Zoladex) are drugs that can be given to suppress the functioning of ovaries and are injections that are given in the muscle. If you are premenopausal, your doctor may use one of these drugs in combination with the tamoxifen and the aromatase inhibitors.

In patients with metastatic breast cancer, hormonal therapies can be given with other treatments to help increase the effectiveness of the drugs. For example, the aromatase inhibitors and fulvestrant can be given with the CDK4/6 inhibitors, and exemestane may be given with evero-limus (see table 4.1, which starts on page 62).

Why Am I on Hormonal Therapy?

If you have an early-stage breast cancer that is hormone receptor–positive, hormonal therapy can be lifesaving. Your doctor will be prescribing these drugs to decrease the risk that the cancer will return. Hormonal therapies can improve your cure rate.

If you have metastatic breast cancer, these drugs can decrease the size of the tumors or keep them stable with the goal of prolonging your life. They can also improve your quality of life even though they won't cure the cancer. Women can be treated with hormonal therapy for long periods of time, sometimes years, before needing to try other treatments, such as chemotherapy.

You should always ask your oncology team why you have been prescribed hormonal therapy. This helps you understand why you need to take your medications as prescribed. If you find it challenging to take your medications, talk to your clinicians about this so they can help you. As an oncologist, I (Jenn) learned early on the importance of being clear about why I am prescribing these medications for patients. Janice is a middle-aged woman with an early-stage hormone receptor–positive breast cancer treated with a lumpectomy and radiation therapy. A couple of months after she finished radiation, I asked how she was doing on anastrozole. "I take it when I remember to take it," she said. "I think of it as a breast health vitamin, so I figured I can take it whenever I remember to take my vitamins." Janice figured that because her tumor had been removed and her breast radiated, she was done with the important part of her treatment.

I reminded Janice that even though her cancer had been physically removed, there might be microscopic cells that have broken off from her initial tumor and entered her bloodstream. This may have happened before she knew she had cancer. The anastrozole would block her body from making the estrogen that could stimulate her cancer cells and cause them to replicate into metastatic cancer. Janice made a plan to put her pill bottle for anastrozole next to her blood pressure medications. Now she tells me she hasn't missed a single dose since that conversation. She even has her daughter bring the pills to her office if she forgets to take one in the morning.

My patient Inez was initially diagnosed with an early-stage breast cancer and was taking anastrozole every day without fail for years. Then she developed a tumor in her hip, which meant that her diagnosis changed to metastatic cancer. I talked with Inez and her husband about the goals of treatment and how they had shifted. While she had been taking hormonal therapy to prevent relapse, now she would take a different hormonal therapy that might help shrink the tumor in her hip and delay the time until the cancer appeared somewhere else. The treatments would reduce her bony pain and hopefully prolong her life.

Remember that there are often several different hormonal treatments to use. Once the cancer progresses on one treatment, there are others we can try. It might be years before we have to start chemotherapy. Inez started taking fulvestrant and palbociclib (a CDK4/6 inhibitor) after this discussion, and she's been doing great on these treatments for more than two years.

Common Side Effects of Hormonal Therapies

While most women do pretty well with hormonal therapy, there are certain common side effects (table 8.1). Some of these side effects may appear in the first few months of therapy but can get better over time—such as hot flashes. Others, such as bone density loss or vaginal dryness, can persist and impact your quality of life throughout your treatment. I always check in with patients about specific side effects because it's hard to take some medication every day if it's making you feel crummy. I also remind people that we have strategies to make these side effects less intrusive on their lives.

Hot Flashes

A hot flash is the sudden sensation of being too warm and is often concentrated in the head, neck, and chest. In some women, this means flushing skin or breaking out in a sudden sweat. Then, as the body cools, you can experience a brief chill. They can happen at any time of day or night, and you may experience hot flashes once a week, once a month, or even hourly. It really varies from person to person.

Table 8.1. Side effects of hormonal treatments and common therapies

Side effect	Behavioral therapies	Other therapies
Hot flashes	Dress in layers, exercise regularly, avoid triggers you have identified (alcohol, certain foods), use fans to cool down	Venlafaxine, some selective serotonin reuptake inhibitors (SSRIs), gabapentin, oxybutynin
Joint stiffness	Regular exercise, yoga	Acupuncture
Vaginal dryness		Over-the-counter vaginal moisturizers for discomfort, vaginal lubricants for intercourse, coconut oil, vitamin E oil, vaginal estrogen (in some cases)
Osteoporosis (loss of bone density)	Dietary calcium (supplements if needed) + vitamin D supplements, weight-bearing exercise, smoking cessation, limited alcohol use	Bisphosphonates (alendronate, e.g., Fosamax; zoledronic acid, e.g., Reclast); RANK ligand inhibitor (denosumab, e.g., Prolia)
Leg cramps	Increase fluid intake, leg stretches, switch timing of hormonal therapy (if taking in the evening, try taking in the morning)	Vitamin B6 supplements, vitamin E supplements, Benadryl
Weight gain	Increase exercise, stick to a healthy diet	
Fatigue	Regular sleep habits; regular exercise	Treat other symptoms (pain, anxiety, hot flashes, depression)
Mood changes	Exercise	Modify hormonal therapy, consider antidepressant therapy

Any of the hormonal therapies can cause these hot flashes, including tamoxifen and the aromatase inhibitors. Menopause also brings on hot flashes, and some women may have been dealing with hot flashes before their breast cancer diagnosis. Women treated with chemotherapy might be pushed into menopause from the infusions, and those who are being treated with leuprolide or goserelin are put into menopause and may also experience hot flashes.

I always ask patients a lot of questions about this side effect. How frequent are the hot flashes? How intense? Do they happen most during the day or at night? Are they preventing you from getting the sleep you need? Once my patient Janice began taking her anastrozole daily after putting it by her blood pressure medication, she started to experience hot flashes, particularly at night. She was waking up sweaty every couple of hours. Her husband described these drenching sweats and said that she needed to change her pajamas each night at least once. Luckily there are some simple lifestyle modifications that may help with hot flashes:

- Dressing in layers allows you to adjust your clothing to your body's changing temperature.
- Identifying and avoiding certain hot flash triggers, such as caffeine, wine, chocolate, or spicy foods.
- Having a fan by your bedside (even if you have air conditioning) can help prevent or decrease the intensity of hot flashes.
- Engaging in regular exercise can help the body regulate its temperature.
- Trying alternative therapies, including acupuncture or meditation, may also be helpful for some women.
- Changing your medication schedule can help. If your hot flashes are at night and you are taking your medication at bedtime, you may try taking it in the mornings instead.

Janice tried several of these techniques and had her daytime hot flashes under control, but she was still pretty miserable at night, despite dressing in layers, turning down the thermostat in her home, and having a fan by her bedside. So we talked about possible medications that could help.

There are medications that are very effective to reduce the burden of hot flashes. Venlafaxine (Effexor) is often prescribed to treat depression and anxiety, but it has also been shown to reduce the frequency of hot flashes. Selective serotonin reuptake inhibitors (SSRIs) such as citalopram (Celexa) and paroxetine (Paxil) have shown to be effective treatments for hot flashes as well. If you are taking tamoxifen, though, it's important to know that some antidepressants (such as paroxetine) will reduce its efficacy, so your doctor will keep this in mind when selecting a hot flash drug for you. Oxybutynin, a medication used for overactive bladder, has been shown in one study to decrease hot flashes in women with breast cancer.

Because Janice didn't really have bothersome hot flashes during the day, I prescribed a low dose of gabapentin at night and that seemed to do the trick. Gabapentin is a drug that is prescribed for several purposes and can be used to treat nerve pain and seizures as well as hot flashes. It is usually prescribed three times a day, but if your hot flashes are most bothersome at night, your doctor may just prescribe it at bedtime. Because it can make you a little drowsy, bedtime dosing may help with both the hot flashes and getting to sleep. Janice's husband even joked that the medication was also helping him get a lot more sleep since she was no longer waking to change her pajamas every night.

There are a lot of over-the-counter supplements or herbs that purport to treat hot flashes. You will want to talk to your doctor before turning to these remedies because they may have estrogenic properties that can counteract your breast cancer therapies. One of my patients with hormone receptor–positive metastatic breast cancer had been taking fulvestrant and palbociclib for almost a year and had been struggling with persistent hot flashes throughout. Katie is a professor of linguistics and described how embarrassing it was to break out into a sweat as she lectured in front of her college students. She cut back on her cups of coffee in the morning and built in more regular exercise, which helped quite a bit, but she still struggled. Katie had been hesitant to add another medication to her list of drugs, so I held off on prescribing something to treat her hot flashes. One day she came in for our appointment and said that she was feeling great with minimal hot flashes. I asked her what had made such a dramatic difference, and she said that she had started taking St. John's Wort. I conferred with my pharmacist, and unfortunately this drug has estrogenic properties and also significantly decreases levels of palbociclib. She was disappointed but open to trying venlafaxine. Once she experienced relief from the hot flashes, she realized that she was willing to take medication to stop them. When I saw her a month later, she was happy to report that her hot flashes remained in check with the venlafaxine.

Joint Stiffness

If you are on an aromatase inhibitor or fulvestrant, your doctor may have discussed the possibility of joint stiffness with you. You may feel stiffness in your muscles and joints after periods of inactivity or when you wake up in the morning. This stiffness often improves with movement and can resolve within minutes of moving around. This is the opposite of arthritic pain, which may worsen throughout the day. Some joint stiffness and muscle aches occur during or after menopause and with age, and it can be hard to sort out if your joint symptoms are directly related to the treatment.

Doctors usually recommend increasing your activity level, and that includes regular exercise. Acupuncture and yoga can sometimes help. You can ask your doctor about whether it's okay to take acetaminophen or ibuprofen as needed, but it is not common to need these medications on a routine basis to treat this type of joint stiffness.

Vaginal Dryness

Postmenopausal women—and those who have entered menopause due to treatment—can experience vaginal symptoms such as dryness and pain with intercourse. The aromatase inhibitors may also contribute to these symptoms. As a first step, I usually recommend over-the-counter vaginal moisturizers and vaginal lubricants. Vaginal moisturizers help with persistent discomfort from vaginal dryness as well as with painful intercourse. They can be applied regularly, usually two or three days per week. Vaginal lubricants, on the other hand, are used at the time of sexual activity. Some women also apply coconut oil or vitamin E to the vulvar region to help with dryness.

If these strategies are not helping, talk to your doctor about whether vaginal estrogens are an option for you. Low doses of estrogen can be delivered to the vaginal region through a vaginal tablet, ring, or cream. In general, the estrogen is delivered locally to the vaginal tissues with very little absorption into the bloodstream. The tablet and the ring tend to have lower rates of absorption than the cream. This is in part because it's difficult to squeeze out a precise dose into the applicator. There are no studies that point to an increased risk of cancer recurrence in women who are using low-dose vaginal estrogens, and if you are bothered by persistent vaginal dryness, talk to your doctor about the possible risks and benefits of vaginal estrogens. If you and your doctor decide to try it, you may be given a low dose for a limited period of time until symptoms improve.

Osteoporosis

Menopause and age are risk factors for osteoporosis, and the aromatase inhibitors may accelerate bone density loss over time. If you are being treated with ovarian suppression and your body is in a temporary menopause, you are also at risk for osteoporosis. Osteoporosis means that you have decreased bone strength and an increased risk of fracture; where osteopenia means that your bones are weaker than normal but not quite at the level of someone with osteoporosis. Even if you have normal bone density now, you may develop osteopenia or osteoporosis over time.

It won't be obvious to you that your bone density is decreasing. Patients sometimes report bone pain or joint pain and wonder if this is caused by the loss of bone density, but this pain is usually caused by something else, such as osteoarthritis. Your doctor may recommend a bone density scan, also called a dual-energy x-ray absorptiometry (DEXA or DXA) scan. The results will help your medical team track your bone density over time. If you are on hormonal therapies that decrease your bone density, your doctor will usually recommend checking a DEXA scan every two years.

There are several lifestyle measures to help reduce bone loss over time, including adequate calcium and vitamin D intake, smoking cessation, and limiting alcohol use. Ideally, it's best to get adequate calcium from your diet alone (1200 mg per day), but if you are getting less than this you may be advised to take calcium supplements. There is some controversy about whether calcium supplements increase the risk of cardiovascular disease, though, so your doctor may encourage you to eat calcium-rich foods instead. Your team may also recommend supplementing with vitamin D because it helps your body to absorb calcium. Some supplements combine vitamin D with calcium, but I often encourage my patients to take them separately so that they can concentrate on getting enough calcium from their diets alone. I also recommend smoking cessation and limiting alcohol to less than one drink per day since both smoking and heavy alcohol use may accelerate bone density loss.

Exercise, as always, is also a great lifestyle measure to take as it has been shown in studies to reduce fracture risk and to even increase bone density. Weight-bearing exercise—such as walking, jogging, jumping, and resistance training—may be particularly helpful. While I don't usually see an increase in bone density from exercise alone, I have some patients who are diligent with regular exercise and have seen improvements in their bone density.

If you have osteoporosis, we usually recommend treatment to prevent further bone density loss and to even help build back some of your bone density. This would be true even if you were not on hormonal therapy. Bone density typically worsens over time and can lead to fractures that can be painful, debilitating, and maybe even require surgery. If you have osteopenia, your doctor may also recommend medications. The bisphosphonates are drugs that help build bone density, and they can be given in pills (alendronate, given weekly) or through an intravenous infusion (zoledronic acid, given every 6 to 12 months). A subcutaneous injection of denosumab may be given every 6 months. Both zoledronic acid and denosumab may also be used to treat bony metastases (chapter 4).

In general, the bisphosphonates are well tolerated, but your doctor will talk to you about the possible side effects. When given intravenously, the bisphosphonates can cause a flu-like reaction for a few days. It occurs more commonly during the first infusion and can often be prevented by taking a dose of acetaminophen prior to treatment. The rare but serious side effects of the bisphosphonates include osteonecrosis of the jaw, which is a condition in which cells in the jaw begin to die. People are usually only at an increased risk if they need major dental work, such as dental extractions. Your doctor may ask you to talk to your dentist before starting these medications and may hold a dose of the medication until any major dental work is done.

That said, the risks of taking bisphosphonates are low and should be balanced with the benefits of preventing fracture. I have a patient in her late fifties with a history of osteopenia, bordering on osteoporosis, who was also taking an aromatase inhibitor for her early-stage breast cancer. Susan was on the beach with her family when she slipped on some rocks and fractured her arm. She needed surgery to repair the fracture and started alendronate when she saw me next. She said that she had initially been hesitant to start a medication for her bones, but after she experienced the pain from a fracture and the subsequent surgery, she wanted to do everything possible to avoid another fracture.

Leg Cramping

Patients who are taking tamoxifen sometimes describe leg cramping that feels like a charley horse. It often occurs in their sleep. While this is uncomfortable and annoying, there are several ways to reduce or prevent this leg cramping. Check the time of day when you are taking your hormonal treatments. If you take them at night, you might switch to taking them in the morning. Dehydration can contribute to leg cramping as well, so drinking plenty of fluids throughout the day can help. Some simple leg stretches for your thighs and calves before bed will also reduce the chance of leg cramping. If this does not work, some experts recommend trying over-the-counter remedies, including vitamin B complex (containing vitamin B6), vitamin E, or diphenhydramine (Benadryl). Some people swear by magnesium supplements, but these have not been shown to be effective in clinical trials. Tonic water, which contains quinine, may be marginally effective but also comes with a small risk of serious cardiac and blood-related side effects.

Weight Changes

Weight gain and loss are reported with almost all of the hormonal therapies, including ovarian suppression (e.g., Lupron), tamoxifen, and the aromatase inhibitors. However, I am usually in discussions with women about their concerns regarding weight gain rather than loss, and it's an important topic to focus on since it's a quality of life issue as well as an overall health issue. As we note in chapter 13, there are often many contributing factors to weight gain, including age over time and menopause, change in activity and/or diet, and the treatments themselves. Whatever the cause may be, the approach to weight management is increasing your physical activity, with a goal of 150 minutes of moderate to vigorous exercise weekly, eating at least five servings of fruits and vegetables daily, and limiting processed foods and alcohol. Gaining weight is frustrating and can negatively impact your quality of life, and your team will want to help you in your efforts to focus on achieving and maintaining a healthy weight.

Fatigue

Feeling tired is a common symptom that patients bring up in an office visit. In women who are taking any hormonal therapy, the question posed to me is often whether I think the fatigue is related to the treatment. There are a lot of variables that contribute to fatigue in all stages of cancer, including sleep disturbances, anxiety, depression, pain, and the treatments themselves. It's important for your team to consider what might be contributing to why you feel so tired and to treat any underlying problems like pain, anxiety, or low mood. If the hormonal therapies are causing hot flashes that are impacting sleep, addressing the hot flashes may help you sleep and therefore increase your energy level. Some of the techniques discussed in chapter 16 can be applied here, particularly exercise and getting a good night's sleep.

Mood Changes

Some women taking ovarian suppression, tamoxifen, or the aromatase inhibitors may experience mood fluctuations or depression. It's sometimes difficult to figure out if this is due to the hormonal therapy or if the mood changes might have happened even without starting hormonal treatments. It's important to be open with your doctor about how you are feeling and whether she thinks it might be related to your treatments. She may talk to you about drug holidays, switching treatments, or strategies to treat depression (see chapter 17).

I just saw Cheryl, a woman in her early thirties with a locally advanced hormone receptor–positive breast cancer, who just completed chemotherapy and started on monthly leuprolide with the plan to add an aromatase inhibitor. After starting leuprolide, she reported big mood swings and had been short-tempered with her husband and kids, which was completely out of character for her. She also reported feeling depressed with no motivation to leave her home or see her friends. She asked whether her symptoms might be due to Lupron. Given the big change in how she was feeling, I recommended holding off on her next Lupron shot, and when she saw me a few weeks later, she was relieved to report that she felt more like herself. She ended up taking tamoxifen without Lupron and has not had any further issues with mood swings or depression.

Other times, I see women who are on hormonal therapies and experience mood changes that may not directly be related to the treatments. If your symptoms are less likely related to the hormonal therapy, your doctor may try different strategies to address these symptoms (see chapter 17).

Taking a Break from Hormonal Treatments

If you and your doctor have tried several strategies to reduce your side effects without luck, talk to your doctor about whether you could take a break from your hormonal treatments. Your doctor may recommend taking a brief break from your medication, perhaps two to four weeks before restarting the drug. This break may help you feel better, while also helping your cancer team figure out what is going on.

Sometimes people take a break from hormonal therapy and restart again with the same drug, only to discover that they have far fewer side effects from it. We don't have a great explanation for why this might happen. It's possible that just taking a brief break from treatment may help you tolerate the therapy better in the long run. Other times, a woman may take a break from hormonal therapy and continue to experience persistent symptoms that do not improve at all. When this happens, I usually recommend connecting with her primary care doctor, since it is possible that something unrelated to breast cancer is causing the symptoms.

One of my patients on anastrozole for an early-stage breast cancer had terrible shoulder pain, particularly in her left shoulder. The pain did not sound typical for the joint pains that women get from hormonal therapy because it lasted all day and was significantly worse with movement, and far worse in her left shoulder as compared to her right shoulder. When she took a break from anastrozole, she was no better. She scheduled a follow-up with her primary care physician, and I also checked a shoulder MRI that showed a big tear in her rotator cuff. Her primary care physician referred her to an orthopedic doctor.

If your symptoms improve during a break and recur after you restart the hormonal therapy, then it's likely that the drug is causing your side effects. Your doctor may talk about trying another drug. Even though the aromatase inhibitors all work in similar ways, your body may be able to tolerate one aromatase inhibitor better than another. This gets a little more complex if you are on hormonal therapies in combination with other targeted therapies for metastatic hormone receptor–positive breast cancer. Sometimes women are experiencing side effects to the treatments added to the hormonal therapies, such as the CDK4/6 inhibitors or mTOR inhibitors. So ask your doctor. There are other strategies to manage this, including reducing dosages.

Rare and Serious Side Effects with Tamoxifen

Although tamoxifen is a very effective drug as hormonal therapy for breast cancer, it also brings the risk of rare but serious side effects in a few women. The first of these is the risk of developing a blood clot, usually in the leg or lungs. People with a blood clot in the leg, also known as a deep vein thrombosis, may experience swelling and discomfort in one calf or foot more than the other. A blood clot in the lungs is called a pulmonary embolus, which can cause shortness of breath or chest pain when you take a deep breath.

People are more at risk for blood clots when they are not as active as they are usually, and this includes long car rides or plane trips, or a planned elective surgery when you may be off your feet for some time. I usually tell patients to take a walk every hour or two if you are on a long plane ride or road trip. If you have an elective surgery planned, you can talk to your team about whether to take a break from tamoxifen for a week before and after your procedure.

Before prescribing tamoxifen, your doctor will review your medical history. If you've experienced a blood clot in the past, your doctor may hold off on treating you with this drug, and if you experience a blood clot while taking tamoxifen, your doctor will probably switch you to something else.

Tamoxifen can also cause irregular menstrual periods, which is not harmful. However, tamoxifen is associated with a low but serious risk of endometrial cancer. For this reason, you will want to let your doctor know if you notice that your periods are more frequent or heavier than normal. It's unlikely that this represents an underlying endometrial cancer, but your team may suggest getting an ultrasound of your uterus or a referral to the gynecology team.

CHAPTER NINE

Controlling Nausea

Everyone associates chemotherapy treatments with nausea. And it might seem that nausea is pretty simple: You feel crummy and you're throwing up. It's awful and you just want someone to do something. In actuality, there are many triggers for nausea or vomiting while you are a cancer patient. And medically, nausea is complicated because it can be triggered by the brain, by the stomach and intestines, by infection, by the medications you are taking, or even by your mood.

Doctors have to consider a lot of factors when treating nausea, and so a colleague came up with a mnemonic (aptly: VOMITING) to help us remember them all. This may sound a little nerdy, but what can you do? When your doctor starts asking a lot of questions about your nausea, you'll know that he or she is thinking along the following lines:

V = Vestibular, meaning anything happening in the brain or inner ear that makes you dizzy.

O = Obstruction, referring to anything in the stomach or colon that may be blocking food from digesting. This includes constipation.

M = Motility, meaning the stomach and intestines aren't pushing food along and it's sitting in your digestive tract.

I = Infection or inflammation, which can be in the stomach or intestines or even in your throat.

T = Toxins, which means any medications you are taking that can cause the side effect of nausea, such as the chemotherapy itself or opioids for pain.

I = Intracranial process, which means nausea can be caused by brain metastases (breast cancer that has spread to the brain).

N = Nerves, meaning anxiety or anticipatory nausea.

G = Gums, mouth, and throat, referring to mouth sores, dry mouth, or a yeast infection in your mouth that can affect your ability or willingness to eat.

With each of these potential causes of nausea comes a different set of techniques to solve the problem, so when you call or come to the clinic and talk about nausea or being unable to eat, your medical team will ask numerous questions to help narrow down the source. If you can give your medical team answers, you will help them find a cause and a solution. Consider the following:

- Do you feel nausea all the time?
- Does eating make the feeling better or worse?
- Is the nausea worse with certain foods? Or after taking certain pills?
- Are you vomiting?
- When you vomit, is it food you ate a while ago? Or is it just a yellow-green fluid (bile)?
- Do you have any heartburn symptoms?
- Are you moving your bowels regularly?
- Do you feel constipated?
- Are you having headaches?
- Have you been able to eat and drink?
- Are you having abdominal pain associated with vomiting?

There are several general categories of causes of nausea. I (Vicki) will describe each one, starting with the most common, and describe the way your doctor may treat it.

Medications That Cause Nausea

As you describe your nausea to your doctor, the first thing he or she will try to rule out is whether it's your medications or treatment that may be the culprit. Almost any medication can cause nausea, but for cancer patients, we know that the most common sources are the cancer therapy itself and the opioids used to treat pain.

Chemotherapy-Induced Nausea

Of course, everyone knows that intravenous chemotherapy can cause nausea. Not all chemotherapies have this side effect, but many of them do. Chemotherapy drugs are thus classified into one of three categories based on their tendency to cause nausea (or vomiting, which is called *emesis*): low emetic risk, moderate emetic risk, and high emetic risk. Depending on the emetic risk of the chemotherapy you are on, your doctor will prescribe the appropriate drug or mix of drugs to reduce or eliminate nausea after infusions, and we have really effective medications to choose from. In general, six classes of antiemetics (anti-vomiting medication) are commonly used to treat nausea caused by chemotherapy (table 9.1). Occasionally we have to go beyond these classes of drugs to control nausea, but thankfully that's a rare event.

Each type of antiemetic uses different mechanisms to prevent nausea, which is why it is safe to use more than one drug at the same time if the doctor thinks that nausea could be a problem on your regimen. Oncologists almost never use two drugs from the same category because they will have overlapping side effects. In general, it's a good idea to ask your oncology team for written instructions on when and how to take all of your antiemetic medications. Your team will tell you which ones to take on a scheduled basis around the time of chemotherapy and which ones you should take only if you have nausea. For people getting chemotherapy regimens with minimal emetic risk, doctors might not prescribe an antinausea drug. For regimens with a low emetic risk, your doctor may

Table 9.1. Six classes of antiemetics

Class	Commonly used medications
Steroids	Dexamethasone (Decadron)
Benzodiazepines	Lorazepam (Ativan)
Dopamine receptor antagonists	Prochlorperazine (Compazine), metoclopramide (Reglan)
5HT3 or serotonin antagonists	Ondansetron (Zofran), granisetron (Kytril), palonosetron (Aloxi)
NK-1 receptor antagonists	Aprepitant (Emend), fosaprepitant (Emend for injection)
Neuroleptics	Olanzapine (Zyprexa)

prescribe you one antiemetic rather than the cocktail of drugs used with chemo regimens that have a higher emetic risk.

Oral Anti-Cancer Drug–Induced Nausea

There are many breast cancer treatments that are given orally. If you have metastatic breast cancer, you might be prescribed targeted therapies used with hormonal therapy (abemaciclib, palbociclib, ribociclib, everolimus). Some anti-HER2 agents (lapatinib, neratinib) and the PARP inhibitors (olaparib, talozaparib) are also oral drugs. There are also oral chemotherapy agents such as capecitabine. Most people don't think pills cause nausea, but some of them can. It's okay to ask your doctor about the possibility of nausea as a side effect when taking any anti-cancer treatment.

Options for Treatment-Related Nausea

5HT3 (Serotonin Receptor) Antagonists

The most common method used to treat chemo-induced nausea is a combination of 5HT3 antagonists and steroids. 5HT3 is a kind of serotonin receptor, and patients may take 5HT3 antagonists, such as ondansetron (Zofran) and palonosetron (Aloxi), prior to getting chemotherapy. Palonosetron is given prior to chemotherapy and actually acts for three more days afterward. Because it is in the same class of medications as ondansetron, you should not take any ondansetron at home until three days have passed since you were given palonosetron.

Ondansetron will work for only eight hours at standard doses. If your doctor prescribes ondansetron prior to chemotherapy, you may be instructed to take this medication every eight hours for three days after your infusion, or you will be advised to take it only as needed. It's important to ask your infusion nurse which 5HT3 antagonist you are receiving and whether you will need to take more of it in the coming days. There are pros and cons to each of the different types.

The 5HT3 antagonists are also used to prevent and treat the nausea from oral anti-cancer drugs. Any nausea and vomiting that persist despite these medications is treated similarly to breakthrough nausea from intravenous chemotherapy. For most people, these drugs manage the nausea effectively. You may not feel much like eating during this time, but you shouldn't feel actively sick.

The primary side effect of 5HT3 antagonists is constipation. Although the safety information about these drugs states that just 5% of patients experience this side effect, most doctors in cancer clinics note that as many as a quarter of all patients can experience constipation. Your doctor may suggest a laxative for you to take if this happens. The reason to treat constipation even if you aren't eating much is that constipation can also cause nausea.

Another side effect that patients may experience with this class of antiemetics is headache. If you notice that you regularly experience a headache each time you take a 5HT3 antagonist, talk to your doctor about whether there may be an alternate antiemetic to try.

Steroids Used with 5HT3 Antagonists

The 5HT3 antagonists often work better when they are given with a steroid, and the most commonly used steroid is dexamethasone. Steroids are safe to take in short episodes, but they can also cause uncomfortable side effects. The most common steroid side effect is a sudden, short burst of energy that lasts for two or three days. People often have trouble sleeping and can be incredibly energetic and creative. I've had husbands and wives complain to me that their spouse is up all night on some type of house project that keeps everyone awake. Then when the effect wears off they can crash and sleep for hours on end.

Steroids may also cause or worsen anxiety and irritability. And the other major side effect of steroids is that they can make your blood glucose run high. If you are diabetic or have a tendency toward high blood sugar, your oncology team may want to monitor your blood sugar levels and may even need to adjust your diabetes medications while you are taking dexamethasone.

You may be wondering why we start with 5HT3 antagonists and steroids if they can cause all of these side effects. The problem with nausea and vomiting is that once it starts it can be very hard to get under control again. Also, most people fear nausea so much when they start chemotherapy that doctors want to keep this side effect under control from the beginning. Many doctors start by prescribing high doses of antinausea medication to make sure that the first chemotherapy cycle goes as smoothly as possible. If it goes well, your doctor may pare down the medication in subsequent cycles until they find the dose that controls your nausea with a minimum of additional side effects. If things don't go smoothly and you are miserable, your oncology team will adjust the medications and make things better.

Yolanda, a 35-year-old woman, was undergoing chemotherapy and anti-HER2 treatments for a stage 3 breast cancer. For the first two chemotherapy treatments she said she was doing okay overall, but when we saw her for her third treatment we noticed that her weight had dropped by almost 10 pounds. Her husband came in for that visit and said she had been experiencing nausea with some vomiting for almost a week after each chemo treatment. Yolanda said, "I expected to feel miserable, so why complain?" She also worried that if she told us how tough the chemo had been, we might decrease the dose or delay the treatment.

It's important to listen to your body and let us know how you are feeling. I tell people to keep a record of their symptoms after the first infusion, how much they ate and drank and how they felt. This is important information to give to the nurses and doctors, who can adjust your medications to make the next infusion easier. Your body is different from everyone else's, and you may react differently to treatment. The point is that you should never feel that you should expect nausea and have to suffer through it. You don't have to feel sick. If you feel nausea after an infusion, contact the clinic right away and tell them how this is affecting your life, because your oncology team or your palliative care clinician can and should prescribe something else to help you.

I always tell my patients that being miserable is never a good plan and that we can always make changes with the goal of helping you feel better while also hopefully keeping you on schedule with your chemo. In Yolanda's case, I added a few additional days of steroids, and she came in for some intravenous fluids a few days after chemotherapy. With these changes, she felt much better, gained a few pounds back, and was able to go back to work while also completing chemotherapy at the full dose and on time.

NK-1 Antagonists

If you are on a chemotherapy regimen that has a high potential to cause nausea, your doctor might prescribe neurokinin-1 (NK-1) receptor antagonists in addition to steroids and 5HT3 antagonists. These drugs can be dramatically effective, so if you experience severe nausea despite taking 5HT3 antagonists and steroids, don't despair. We've had many patients successfully control nausea when we add one of these medications.

Neuroleptics

Olanzapine is an antipsychotic medication that is also very effective at treating nausea from chemotherapy. It blocks several receptors in the brain, including dopamine receptors and serotonin receptors. Your doctor may use this medication as part of a standard antiemetic regimen prior to chemotherapy and for a few days afterward, or she may add this medication if your current regimen is not working effectively.

Patients often express concern about being treated with a drug in the antipsychotic family. One patient who had been a nurse for decades recognized the drug name and initially refused to take it, even though she was really struggling with nausea after each infusion. I told her that olanzapine has been studied in many clinical trials with cancer patients and is very effective. She decided to give it a try and said that she was pleasantly surprised at how much better she felt after the next infusion. This medication can cause mild short-term sedation, but this can be helpful for some patients who are taking it at night.

Other Medications

A few patients have nausea despite these medications, and we call this breakthrough nausea, because it breaks through the antiemetics. Don't give up if you experience some breakthrough nausea. Your doctor can still prescribe something to help. In this case, you might be given prochlorperazine (Compazine) or lorazepam (Ativan) for additional help. These other two classes of agents, dopamine receptor antagonists and benzodiazepines, are typically used for the occasional breakthrough nausea, and they can be particularly effective in specific circumstances. For instance, lorazepam is a great drug for anticipatory nausea, which is a type of nausea that some people feel when they are just walking into the hospital or infusion unit. It's possible that the mere thought of getting the chemotherapy or the smell of a hospital will make a few people nauseated. Benzodiazepines are also very effective at preventing this type of nausea.

The other benefit of lorazepam is that you don't have to swallow it. Instead, you can let it melt under your tongue. Sometimes, I get calls at night from patients whose antinausea medication has worn off. Their nausea prevents them from swallowing any pills to help. I tell them to put a lorazepam tablet under their tongue and let it melt. In fifteen minutes, they feel well enough to swallow their other antinausea medications.

Cannabinoids and Medical Marijuana

Cannabinoids are the chemicals in marijuana that cause drug-like effects. Dronabinol is a cannabinoid that is approved by the US Food and Drug Administration for the treatment of nausea and vomiting from chemotherapy that breaks through the standard antinausea medications. This medication can have side effects that include dry mouth, fatigue, drowsiness, confusion, or a feeling of euphoria.

There is a lot of interest in using medical marijuana to treat the symptoms related to cancer, including nausea and vomiting. Tetrahydrocannabinol (THC) and cannabidiol (CBD) are two of the most studied chemicals in marijuana and are found in different levels in different strains of marijuana. Medical marijuana comes in several different formulations, including edibles, oils, creams, sprays, and vape pens. Most dispensaries also offer dried leaves or buds for smoking. The research on medical marijuana is limited, and it can contribute its own side effects, such as dizziness, increased heart rate, low blood pressure, hallucinations, and paranoia.

In clinic, I notice that patients who have some prior experience with marijuana and its effects do well with it as a treatment for various cancer treatment side effects, including nausea. Those with little or no experience are sometimes disoriented by these effects. Everyone is different. If you live in a state that has legalized medical marijuana, you should talk to your doctor about whether this might be helpful for you. Most medical marijuana dispensaries are staffed by people who can offer great advice about the different formulations to help target nausea and vomiting.

Integrative Therapies

There are pressure points on the body that can be stimulated to reduce symptoms such as inflammation, pain, and nausea. Acupressure uses pressure on the skin to this effect, and acupuncture uses fine needles. With electroacupuncture, a therapist allows a small electrical current to pass through the acupuncture needles.

There is no strong clinical trial data yet to support the use of these techniques for nausea, though the guidelines published by the American Society of Clinical Oncology do support the use of acupressure and electroacupuncture as an addition to antiemetics. Some chemotherapy infusion suites may even offer acupuncture or Reiki (which uses acupressure points) during chemotherapy sessions.

The addition of ginger to conventional antinausea regimens has been studied in clinical trials with mixed results, and some guidelines support its use in addition to standard antiemetics.

Staying Ahead of Chemo-Induced Nausea

Many times, patients think they should take antiemetic medications only after they start to feel crummy, but your doctor may recommend taking them around the clock for the first two or three days of a chemotherapy cycle to get the full benefit. Other patients stop taking them too soon, and then they start to feel sick, at which point the medication needs time to take effect again once it's restarted. It's much easier to stay ahead of nausea than to play catch-up once the nausea starts. That's why doctors are often insistent that patients take medications to prevent nausea even if they aren't feeling sick.

You should expect that any chemo-induced nausea will be well controlled, although it may take a little bit of trial and error with your oncology team. Here's what you can to do help:

- Take your antiemetics exactly as prescribed.
- If your team has given you a regimen that needs to be taken on a scheduled basis (around the clock), do it. Don't wait for nausea to start. The goal is to prevent the nausea from coming on at all.
- Tell your team if the regimen they prescribed is not working. There are other options.
- Don't let yourself get dehydrated. Keep drinking water, even if you don't feel like eating.
- If you are having real trouble keeping fluids down, you might need to come in to the infusion center to get some IV fluids.
- If your team is having a tough time managing the nausea, ask for a palliative care consult.

Opioid-Induced Nausea and Its Treatment

Opioids are the medications your doctor may prescribe to help with pain. They do a great job of controlling pain, but they have the unfortunate side effect of causing nausea in two different ways. They can directly affect parts of your brain responsible for nausea, such as the chemoreceptor trigger zone and the vomiting center. They also can cause your digestion to slow down, which results in constipation that can eventually lead to nausea. Some people experience nausea in the first few days of starting the medication. For most patients the nausea goes away after those first three to five days. We just need to treat the nausea with effective medications until the body gets used to the pain medication. Dopamine antagonists such as prochlorperazine (Compazine) can be quite effective, and your doctor may recommend you take this every six to eight hours as needed in those first few days. Some patients react differently to different opioids. So for example, morphine may cause nausea in one person but not in another, and the same is true for oxycodone, hydromorphone, and fentanyl.

Cindy was a patient being treated with hormonal therapies for her hormone receptor-positive breast cancer. When she developed metastases in her bones, I prescribed a low dose of opioids to help manage the pain, and they seemed to work well. A couple of weeks later, Cindy told me that her pain had become so distracting that it was hard for her to sleep at night, which made it impossible to function at work. Initially, I became concerned that the cancer might be getting worse and planned to talk to her oncologist about the worsening pain. Cindy then told me that she had stopped taking opioids because they made her so queasy. She would take one at night and then just lie awake feeling sick. We restarted the opioids and added some prochlorperazine as needed, and she started feeling back to her baseline soon after.

In most cases, your body gets used to pain medication, and the nausea goes away after the first few days. Talk to your doctor about the possibility that pain medication may be causing your nausea. You might have to take a lower dose at first or start an anti-nausea medicine like we did with Cindy.

Also remember to take laxatives to treat the constipation caused by the opioids, even after the first few days. Constipation is the most common side effect of opioids and does not go away. As long as you are on opioids, you will probably need to take laxatives (what doctors sometimes call a "bowel regimen") every day.

Gastrointestinal Causes of Nausea and Related Treatments

In addition to the more common causes discussed so far, nausea can also result from some kind of mechanical problem in the gastrointestinal (GI) tract. All of your digestion takes place in what is essentially a long tube that runs from your mouth through the esophagus, stomach, intestines, and to the rectum. Your body moves food along through a series of involuntary muscle contractions, so nutrients and waste are pushed from one section of the GI tract to the next. Any number of factors can interfere with this process and back up the system, which in turn can cause nausea.

Gastroparesis

This is a common cause of nausea, particularly when the feeling of nausea is constant. Gastroparesis is a technical term that means your stomach isn't emptying of food. Everything you have eaten is sort of just sitting there because the stomach isn't contracting enough to move it into the intestines, and after a while your stomach signals the nausea centers in your brain that something is wrong.

There are several reasons this may be happening. Sometimes pain medications, such as opioids, slow the activity in the GI tract. Sometimes you might have severe constipation, and if the intestines can't empty, the stomach can't either. Less commonly, there might be a tumor in the intestines or stomach that is interfering with digestion.

You can suspect gastroparesis if your nausea is pretty much constant and if you are vomiting food you have eaten hours before. Your doctor will be looking for an underlying cause of this nausea, but the ultimate goal is to get the food moving again so that you feel better. Metoclopramide (Reglan) is a medication that stimulates motility in the GI tract and can help with the nausea caused by gastroparesis. Note that your doctor is going to ask about your bowel movements as well, because they want to make sure to treat any underlying constipation that may be contributing to your stomach troubles as well.

Constipation

This is the most common cause of nausea after chemotherapy-induced nausea. If you've been in treatment any length of time and have been taking antiemetics or opioids for pain, you probably know about constipation (see chapter 10). If your constipation is bad enough to cause general nausea, you probably need to adjust your dose of laxatives or the frequency with which you take them. Don't be afraid to bring this up with your doctor. Helping you get this under control should be a priority for your medical team. Some patients choose to reduce the antiemetics they take after a chemotherapy infusion because they would rather endure short-term nausea than deal with constipation that makes them feel crummy later. This is a trade-off that you can make as a patient.

Heartburn

You may or may not have struggled with heartburn or acid reflux in the past, but sometimes this symptom flares up during treatment and may lead to feeling queasy or sick to your stomach. Heartburn can also be a side effect of the steroids that may be used with chemotherapy. Sometimes treating acid reflux may help with nausea, and your doctor may recommend a trial of acid reflux medications, such as histamine-2 receptor antagonists (ranitidine or famotidine) or proton pump inhibitors (omeprazole or pantoprazole). You may also try avoiding some foods that cause heartburn, including spicy or fatty foods, citrus, tomatoes, chocolate, mints, caffeine, and alcohol.

Abdominal Tumors

As cancer progresses, you can develop tumors in the lining of the abdomen, called peritoneal carcinomatosis. The peritoneum is a thin membrane that covers the organs in the abdomen. Sometimes a tumor will metastasize to the membrane and cause the bowels to function erratically. It can look like a spider web growing over the intestines, making it difficult for them to move effectively, which in turn causes nausea and bloating. The best treatment for this is treating the cancer itself. It's also very important to have any underlying constipation under control because constipation will make the symptoms from peritoneal carcinomatosis worse.

Liver Dysfunction

The liver's job is to rid the body of toxins. If the liver is having trouble functioning, these toxins may build up and cause nausea. Also, if you have tumors growing in the liver, they can affect the way the stomach pushes food through to the intestines, meaning that liver tumors can contribute to gastroparesis. If it's not possible to treat the underlying cause of liver dysfunction, you can ask your doctor about the possibility of taking antinausea medications. Remember that you may need to take them at a lower dose than normal if your liver is having trouble metabolizing medications.

Neurologic Causes of Nausea and Its Treatment

Your brain contains receptors that help coordinate and initiate the act of vomiting. This is a safety measure that helps the body rid the stomach of toxins. So you can imagine that anything that affects your brain, or the vestibular nerve (which regulates balance), can cause you to feel or be sick. A metastasis in your brain can cause swelling that increases the pressure in these nausea centers and make you feel sick. If this is the case, you will probably—but not always—experience a headache as well. If you have nausea along with a headache, you need to alert your oncology team. Often doctors will prescribe steroids to decrease the swelling in the brain. You may also need radiation or surgery to treat the tumors.

A patient's son paged me the day after Thanksgiving to let me know that his mother, Mariela, had been experiencing more persistent nausea and had not been able to eat her Thanksgiving meal, which was so unlike her. When I called her, she told me she had also experienced headaches and balance difficulties all week. I called the oncologist right away, and she ordered a brain scan that day that showed a new metastasis causing her symptoms. Mariela started on steroids and was seen by the radiation oncologist who prescribed a short course of radiation. Her nausea, headaches, and balance difficulties improved with treatment, and she started back on breast cancer therapies after completing radiation.

Sensory Causes of Nausea

All different kinds of sensory inputs can induce nausea. Some of my patients will be doing fine and then smell something that triggers an intense reaction. It might be the smell or sight of food, even foods they had previously loved. Chemotherapy can cause short-term nausea after an infusion, but it can also cause a low-grade nausea that is sensitive to strong smells. It's sort of like being pregnant and having a reaction to certain kinds of smells. Remember that this usually won't last forever.

I had a patient who prided herself on cooking delicious meals for her family. Every week the whole extended family would gather at her house to eat her elaborate meals and spend time together. Her daughters described beloved recipes passed down from their grandmother and mother. While being treated with chemotherapy, the smell of her favorite foods made her queasy, and it became impossible for her to cook. She was really saddened by this interruption in family tradition, but her daughters arranged a weekly potluck so she could still enjoy seeing everyone and could choose foods that were more appetizing to her palate. When this same patient switched to a new line of chemotherapy, the queasy feeling went away, and she was able to get back into the kitchen.

So you may need to avoid certain foods while you are in a certain chemotherapy regimen and look for other foods that are more appealing. Trust your body and be kind to yourself while you are getting through this time. You may want to drink smoothies or protein supplement drinks if you need to. Many people find that eating smaller meals more frequently can be a good strategy. You may find that you need really small portions at first. A whole muffin might be overwhelming, so start with a half or a quarter and work your way up.

Anxiety

Have you ever had a feeling of anxiety that was so intense that you actually felt sick to your stomach? If the answer is yes, that's because anxiety can cause nausea, and if you are feeling anxious during treatment or if you are having trouble with issues not related to treatment, these feelings can create or exacerbate nausea.

If you don't want to take antianxiety medications to treat anxiety, you can look into cognitive behavioral therapy (a form of psychotherapy in which the patient works with a therapist on the interaction of thoughts and behaviors on feelings; see chapter 12) and get some techniques for calming down during stressful times. But anxiety can also be treated effectively with a low dose of lorazepam (Ativan) or olanzapine (Zyprexa). Lorazepam can cause confusion in some people, however, and in that case olanzapine may be a better choice.

Belinda is a patient with hormone receptor–positive metastatic breast cancer who has been treated with several types of hormonal therapy, clinical trials, and chemotherapy. After scans showed that her tumor had progressed, she switched chemotherapies, and she did well on the treatments with minimal side effects. Then the infusion nurse called me to say that Belinda was experiencing bothersome nausea and was also really anxious about her upcoming scans. When I asked Belinda about this in clinic, she said she had been feeling nervous for several weeks about her scans and that her nausea was most prominent when her mind was racing. We both thought that the underlying cause of her nausea was likely anxiety, and she tried olanzapine, which worked really well for both symptoms.

* * *

Nausea is a blanket term that covers a lot of possible causes, and treating nausea requires ongoing interaction with your medical team. It's important to tell the clinicians about your nausea whenever it occurs. This is one of those symptoms, like pain, in which you need to be proactive with your medical team because they have tools to help you and they want you to feel your best.

CHAPTER TEN

Managing Constipation and Diarrhea

Bowel movements are a popular subject with oncologists. This is because some cancer therapies may cause diarrhea, while a few others can cause constipation. On top of this, many of the medications we prescribe to treat nausea and pain can cause constipation. You may experience both constipation and diarrhea during the course of treatment, and your medical team will be checking in with you about changes in your bowel function as a result. Don't worry. Your doctor has a lot of strategies to use to treat both of these conditions and help you feel more comfortable.

How the GI Tract Works

Doctors take the unromantic view of the gastrointestinal tract as a long hose that handles intake at the mouth and esophagus, processes nutrition in the stomach and small intestine, and eliminates waste through the colon, rectum, and anus (figure 10.1). We also think of the movement of food, nutrition, and waste as a transit system. This transit is managed by muscular contractions, called peristalsis, in the wall of the GI tract. You may be able to feel how the esophagus pushes food down into your stomach; the stomach and intestines also push food along with similar contractions. So does the colon and rectum.

Peristalsis is governed by a complex system of nerves that are autonomic, meaning that you don't have any voluntary control over them. Doctors are only beginning to understand this GI nervous system—sometimes called the enteric nervous system—and all the ways in which it works to regulate digestion and even hunger. We do know that it is connected through a series of hormones to the central nervous system. It consists of about five hundred million neurons, many more than you have in your spinal cord.

There are numerous ways that cancer and cancer treatment can affect the enteric nervous system and the body's ability to regulate digestion. Many chemotherapy regimens affect the cells lining the intestines and increase transit time in the bowels, which leads to diarrhea. Other medications that treat pain and chemo-induced nausea often have the side effect of slowing down peristalsis throughout the GI tract or in the lower bowels specifically. This can cause sudden and severe constipation.

People sometimes think that they can regulate their bowels through diet alone. Diet does matter, and foods such as chocolate and pizza can be very constipating, while diets rich in fiber from grains and salads can

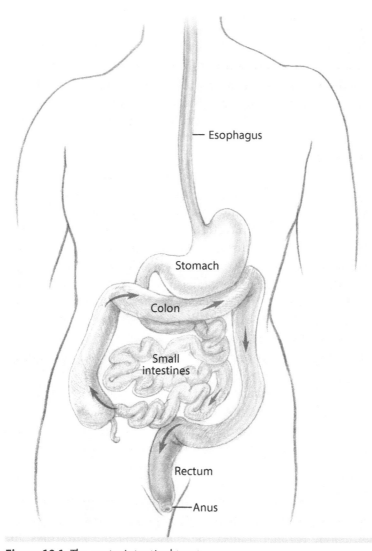

Figure 10.1. The gastrointestinal tract

increase the rate at which stool goes through the GI tract. So if you have constipation or diarrhea caused by treatment or medication, certain dietary choices can make the situation better or worse. The problem is that medications can have powerful effects on how your bowels function, and it's almost impossible to counteract these effects through diet alone.

Cycling between Constipation and Diarrhea

Regulating your bowels during chemotherapy treatment can be tricky for some people. People taking antiemetics (antinausea drugs) may have constipation for the first week after an infusion. Then in the second week, when they have stopped taking the antiemetics, they may experience diarrhea from the chemotherapy itself. Toggling between constipation and diarrhea like this can be very frustrating, and figuring out a short course of laxatives that works well can take time.

I (Dave) always tell my patients that we probably can't make it perfect, but we can make the situation livable. Treating constipation is often more art than science, and it may take several infusions for your medical team to get a handle on things. I also ask patients to tell me which side effect they fear more, the constipation or the diarrhea. Most people who have experienced both say that they don't like diarrhea but that they truly hate constipation. When you are constipated, you often feel more uncomfortable. Many people don't feel like doing anything and they don't feel social. By contrast, while diarrhea is never pleasant, it isn't painful, and most people can function pretty well between episodes.

Signs of Constipation

Everyone who has experienced constipation knows the telltale signs of feeling bloated, maybe feeling discomfort in the bowels or cramping in the lower abdomen. Even if you don't feel these symptoms, you may want to be aware of some other signs of constipation and bring them up with your medical team:

- Not having a regular bowel movement, every day or every other day, if you did so before starting cancer treatment.
- Failing to move your bowels for three to five days. Even if you aren't having pain, you may need treatment for constipation.

- Small stools that are difficult to pass. They can be hard pellets of stool. Patients sometimes tell me that they go every day, but the colon can still get backed up if you aren't producing enough stool.
- Straining to produce stool. This can be an early warning sign of constipation.
- Abdominal pain or cramping.
- Swollen or distended abdomen as the large intestine becomes impacted, or blocked with stool.
- Nausea or vomiting. If your colon is backed up, the food in your stomach has no place to go.
- In severe cases, patients will say that they have liquid stool or diarrhea when they are in fact constipated. The reason is that only liquid can get around the hard, impacted stool in the left side of the colon.

Constipation Caused by Medications or Treatment

If you develop constipation, your doctor will be thinking right away that certain medications and conditions of treatment are a likely culprit:

- Opioids for pain
- Antinausea medications, particularly the 5HT3 antagonists, such as ondansetron (Zofran), palonosetron (Aloxi), and granisetron (Kytril)
- Some chemotherapies
- Aluminum-containing antacids such as Maalox
- Dehydration due to treatment

Most doctors will warn people about constipation, but many people have had no experience with serious constipation before they start cancer treatment. If you've ever been prescribed opioids for pain after a surgery, then you may understand what kind of effect these drugs can have on your bowels. The constipation caused by antinausea medications and opioids can be severe.

Opioids

Nearly everyone who takes an opioid for pain relief will experience constipation. The GI tract has an independent system of active neurons, like those found in the brain and spinal cord. These contain opioid receptors, and when an opioid binds with them, they slow down the contraction and relaxation phases of peristalsis, and that slows down the whole transit system that's moving food and waste through your body. This includes the anal sphincter, which may be less able to relax enough to let stool pass easily. These opioids also affect the way the body absorbs fluid in the intestines, further making stools dehydrated and harder.

This is why your doctor will almost always give you a recommendation for a laxative alongside the opioid and tell you to start taking the two at the same time. Nobody likes to take extra pills, and some patients claim that they have had good luck with using prune juice or other home-remedy laxatives in their past encounters with constipation. But in many years of treating cancer patients, I've found that these natural remedies that may have worked in the past don't usually work as well with opioid-induced constipation. With this kind of constipation, adding fiber to your diet can make stool rock-like and still not move it, so we usually don't recommend fiber drinks or supplements. It's better to treat this side effect seriously from the beginning with a scheduled laxative.

My patient Indira started taking a long-acting opioid to control the pain from a small tumor in her hip bone. At first, she was diligent about taking a laxative alongside the pain medication. About a month later, she came to the clinic complaining of bloating and constipation. We figured out that she had become much more active and busy once her pain was under better control. As a result, she had forgotten to take the laxatives. Once she added them back into her daily regimen, her bowels got back on track. Troubleshooting isn't always as straightforward as this, but for many people a scheduled laxative regimen—what doctors call a bowel regimen—works well.

Antinausea Medications

The second major cause of constipation that we see is from the antinausea medications that you take when you get chemotherapy, particularly the 5HT3 antagonists, such as ondansetron and granisetron. Jenn had a patient named Elisa who was 43 when she started neoadjuvant chemotherapy for an early-stage breast cancer. After the first cycle of chemotherapy, Elisa experienced constipation from the antinausea medication ondansetron. When she saw her medical team before her next cycle, we recommended a scheduled laxative regimen. Instead, she tried prunes and some tea that she said had worked for her in the past. Unfortunately, the constipation got so bad that she developed anal fissures, which are sort of like paper cuts in the anus. Elisa said that the pain from the fissures was far worse than any of the side effects of her chemotherapy. Jenn referred her to a rectal surgeon who got her started on some extra medications to heal the fissures, and then she started on a regular bowel regimen to help prevent constipation through her remaining cycles.

If you are experiencing constipation from the antinausea medications, there are some simple things you can do to try to prevent and treat the constipation. First, try starting your laxatives the day before chemotherapy. You want to prime the pump. Second, continue your laxative for one day beyond your final dose of the antinausea drug that is causing the constipation. So if you are taking an antinausea medication for three days, you'll need the laxative for four days. Your doctor will usually recommend taking a medication like polyethylene glycol (Miralax) or senna, which will be described in more detail later.

Some Chemotherapies

While in treatment with chemotherapy, you might become constipated. This is often caused by the other medications you are taking for pain (opioids) or to prevent nausea (5H3T antagonists). It might also be caused by the chemotherapy itself in some cases. Certain therapies for breast cancer are known to cause constipation, including vinorelbine (Navelbine) and eribulin (Halaven). Your oncologist will know which chemotherapy regimens cause constipation and will prescribe something to treat it.

Aluminum-Containing Antacids

Certain over-the-counter medications can also contribute to constipation, particularly those used to treat stomach acid and acid reflux. I know of one patient who reported that her chemotherapy regimen was causing heartburn. Her doctor couldn't figure out why her constipation was so hard to control, until the patient reported that she was swallowing nearly a bottle of Maalox in the days following every infusion. The active ingredient in Maalox is aluminum hydroxide, which neutralizes gastric acids but also causes constipation. She switched to a different antacid, milk of magnesia, with the active ingredient of magnesium hydroxide, which also neutralizes stomach acid but more often causes loose stools. That small change made all the difference.

Dehydration

The known side effects from both cancer and treatment include nausea, loss of appetite, and bowel trouble. Each one of these can contribute to dehydration. The less you eat and drink, the more your GI tract will struggle to work well. The function of the colon is to resorb water from the GI tract, and one of the ways that we preserve water when we are dehydrated is increased absorption of water through the colon. So dehydration can lead to a terrible cycle of constipation, where patients don't feel like eating and drinking because they get constipated, which in turn leads to more constipation. That's why your doctors and nurse practitioners will constantly be reminding you to drink water.

Jenn is treating Giana, a young woman in her thirties, with neoadjuvant chemotherapy, and she had been experiencing some constipation that I think was related to dehydration. She told us that she was keeping up with her food and water intake, but when her husband came to her last visit, he said she had been experiencing some mild nausea and didn't feel like eating or drinking much. Giana said she was so busy keeping up with their toddler and trying to put in some hours at work that she hadn't bothered taking any antinausea medications; she didn't think the nausea was that bad. After she tried antinausea medication, however, she felt more inclined to eat and drink, and her bowels became more regular. She still uses an occasional laxative but hasn't needed it on a scheduled basis.

Older patients may be at high risk for developing dehydration because they are more susceptible to the side effects of minor dehydration, and often their kidney function is not as robust. Your medical team will be urging you to continue to drink fluids even if you aren't hungry and to try to take small meals throughout the day to combat dehydration.

Feeling Constipated, Even When You Aren't

It's possible to have a bloated feeling or a sensation of cramps even though you are passing soft stools or even loose stools every day. It's tempting to describe that feeling as the feeling of being constipated. Sometimes people aren't constipated in the strict sense of the word, but their brain is telling them otherwise because the cancer is making them feel this way. Some cancer-related conditions, such as peritoneal carcinomatosis (abdominal tumors), can contribute to the feeling of constipation. Others, such as hypercalcemia and hypothyroidism, actually cause constipation.

Peritoneal Carcinomatosis

The peritoneum is a very thin membrane that lines the abdomen and covers the organs inside it. Peritoneal carcinomatosis is a form of metastatic spread when the breast cancer disseminates into the peritoneum throughout your abdomen in little nodules that I often compare to sand or sugar granules. The nodules can eventually grow together and form large clumps of tumor that wrap around the bowels. The presence of these multiple small metastases throughout the abdomen can actually slow down the movement of the bowel, leading to constipation. But just the presence of metastases in the abdomen can activate nerve endings that tell the brain that you are constipated even though you may not actually have any stool in your colon. The presence of tumor nodules can displace these nerves and also cause dysfunctional communication between parts of the nervous system that regulates bowel movement.

Hypercalcemia

This is a condition in which your body has unusually high levels of calcium. Cancer patients are at risk for hypercalcemia for multiple reasons. They could have bone metastases, or their cancer cells can produce a substance that mimics the parathyroid hormone, the hormone that regulates calcium. When they get dehydrated from hypercalcemia, they get constipated.

Karen has hormone receptor–positive metastatic breast cancer that has spread to the bones. She initially declined cancer therapies for about a year but came back to see our team after she experienced increasing bone pain and constipation. Her tumor had progressed quite a bit in her bones, and her calcium level was very elevated. She started on hormonal therapy and a bisphosphonate, and her pain and calcium level decreased over time and have normalized. Her constipation improved, too, so I think that it was at least due in part to the elevated calcium levels she had been experiencing previously.

Treating Constipation

If your constipation is caused by the cancer itself, the best way to treat it is by treating the cancer with the systemic therapies that we talked about in chapter 4. Your doctor will likely also prescribe medications to improve stool transit in the short term, until the cancer treatment takes effect.

If your constipation is more likely caused by medication used in your cancer treatment, your doctor will prescribe a bowel regimen of laxatives, the most common of which are listed in table 10.1. Again, treating con-

Table 10.1. Laxatives by strength and mechanisms

Strength and type	Mechanism of action
Mild	
Fruits and vegetables	Bulking agent
Fiber (Metamucil, Citrucel, Benefiber, etc.)	Bulking agent (causes gas)
Docusate (Colace)	Emollient (wets and softens stool)
Bisacodyl (Dulcolax)	Stimulant
Moderate	
Magnesium hydroxide (Milk of Magnesia)	Hyperosmotic (draws water into the bowels)
Polyethylene glycol (Miralax)	Hyperosmotic
Senna (Ex-Lax, Senokot)	Stimulant
Strong	
Lactulose	Hyperosmotic
Magnesium citrate	Hyperosmotic
Naloxone, methylnaltrexone (Relistor)	Opioid antagonist

stipation is more art than science, and your doctor will give you guidance on how and when to use these medications safely. Several major classes of laxatives that doctors use in breast cancer treatment are described in more detail here.

Osmotic Laxatives

One of the mainstays of treatment in the cancer clinic, osmotic laxatives work by holding more water within the intestinal tract and also drawing water into the GI tract. These medications can make stools a little watery, almost like diarrhea, but patients can easily modify the dose by how loose their stools are. They are extremely effective against constipation from opioids and the antinausea medications like the 5HT3 antagonists. We often recommend that patients start an osmotic laxative prior to using opioids or antinausea medications.

One example of a commonly used osmotic agent is polyethylene glycol (Miralax). This is the same substance that is used in most colonoscopy preps, but rest assured, you will be taking a much lower dose. Remember that to take it effectively, you have to drink four to six ounces of water, and this can be difficult for people who are nauseated. Sometimes your doctor may recommend taking this up to twice daily. If you have difficulty taking Miralax, ask your doctor about an alternative osmotic laxative or adding stimulant laxatives, which come in pill form.

Other osmotic laxative options include milk of magnesia. You can take two tablespoons (30cc) every six hours, and this will often start the bowels moving and relieve constipation. Your doctor can also prescribe lactulose, which is a synthetic sugar that causes the colon to retain fluid. It's syrupy sweet, and some patients don't like it because it's so sweet. Magnesium citrate, a saline laxative, is also an osmotic, and a full glass of magnesium citrate usually induces a bowel movement.

The process of learning how to control constipation is individual, and you will have to experiment. The osmotic agents are often effective, but they can be difficult to titrate with cancer therapies and opioids, and thus patients can swing into a day or two of diarrhea. If you get diarrhea from these agents, stop taking them for 12 to 24 hours or until the diarrhea goes away. If you are on opioids, your medical team will probably tell you to start them again after going 24 hours without a bowel movement.

Stimulants

These drugs help move stool through the intestines by activating the enteric nervous system and stimulating the bowels. Senna (Ex-Lax) and bisacodyl (Dulcolax) are examples of stimulant laxatives. These drugs, along with osmotic laxatives, are key to treating constipation in patients with cancer. And remember that you might need a higher dose than the package recommends.

Many patients tell me that they stopped taking senna because it didn't work. When I ask how much they were taking, it's usually one or two tablets per day (most over-the-counter tablets are 8.6 milligrams each). Others may have taken it a few times, but skipped it on other days. I usually have people re-try it on a daily, scheduled basis and increase the dose if needed (you can take up to 68.8 milligrams of senna per day). This often does the trick to get things moving. The stimulants are a nice option to treat constipation because they are tablets, which are a lot more convenient, especially if you are out and about and don't want to fiddle with mixing your Miralax with a glass of water.

Opioid Antagonists

For patients on opioids, naloxone can be a very effective drug for treating constipation. Naloxone competes with such opioids as hydromorphone, morphine, and oxycodone at the opioid receptors and blocks the effects of the opioids. In higher doses, emergency responders use it intravenously to counteract effects of an opioid drug overdose. When taken orally at low doses, it is not absorbed into the system. Instead, it blocks the opioid receptors in the intestinal tract alone. This is a great help to cancer patients taking opioids for pain because it doesn't block the opioid receptors anywhere in the body except in the GI tract. So your pain medication will still treat the cancer pain, but your stomach and intestines will be free to digest food as usual.

Naloxone is unpleasant to take orally, and so an injection under the skin called methylnaltrexone (Relistor) was created to make it easier to use. This medication is typically given every other day, although some patients don't like to get an injection that often. You should also know that most insurance companies won't cover Relistor unless the patient has tried all the other laxatives and they have not been effective.

Emollients

An emollient is a softening agent, and these bowel medications are often called stool softeners. An emollient laxative draws more fats and water into the stool and makes them easier to pass. The most common example is docusate (Colace). If you take an emollient, you'll notice that your stools will become softer and more liquid. This kind of laxative can be helpful for patients who have anal fissures or hemorrhoids that can be irritated by hard stools.

And although these medications may be effective for mild constipation, emollients will rarely be prescribed as the sole laxative to treat constipation caused by opioids or antinausea medications. In fact, one study found no benefit to adding docusate to senna for patients with opioid-induced constipation. However, you can consider adding a stool softener as a second laxative when stools are hard or dry. Vicki often tells patients that emollients create "mush without push," which is why they aren't as useful as other laxatives.

Emollients can also be given as enemas, such as a soap suds enema. These are often difficult for cancer patients to self-administer, but nurses may do this for patients in the hospital or other assisted-living environments.

Can I Just Increase My Fiber?

People often ask about using fiber to treat constipation. Over-the-counter fiber supplements normally work by bulking up the stool to help move it along the intestinal tract. Examples include Metamucil, Citrucel, and Benefiber. Prior to being diagnosed with cancer, these supplements may have been your go-to approach for regulating the bowels. However, the constipation that you may experience with cancer and cancer therapies are usually treated more effectively with the other strategies just outlined. It is also important to note that fiber is not recommended to treat constipation caused by opioids.

Diarrhea

The opposite of constipation is diarrhea, and nearly everyone knows what that's like. But when a physician or nurse practitioner in the cancer clinic asks you whether you are having diarrhea, what they are really asking is whether you have had any increase in bowel movements. These don't need to be the kind of liquid stools people often associate with stomach flu or food poisoning. In fact, they can be semisolid or loose or liquid.

Different cancer treatments can cause diarrhea, including some intravenous chemotherapies, oral chemotherapy (capecitabine), and HER2-targeted therapies (pertuzumab, neratinib, lapatinib). This is also true of some drugs used in hormone receptor–positive metastatic breast cancer (abemaciclib, alpelisib). Patients are sometimes surprised by how quickly they can move from the constipation caused by antinausea medications to the diarrhea caused by the cancer therapies, and it can take a couple of cycles for us to figure out the best course of medications to prevent these swings. Other various causes of diarrhea to be aware of are given in table 10.2.

Jenn has a 76-year-old patient who started on letrozole and abemaciclib to treat a hormone receptor–positive breast cancer with bone and lung metastases. The patient is an avid golfer who had a standing weekly tee time with her buddies. By far the most bothersome side effect of her treatment had been the unpredictable diarrhea. She was missing her golf dates because she felt she needed to be close to a bathroom and felt embarrassed by the frequent, urgent bowel movements. She ended up taking loperamide (Imodium) in the mornings on a scheduled basis, and

Table 10.2. Major causes of diarrhea

Cause	Examples
Traditional chemotherapy	Capecitabine (Xeloda)
HER2-targeted agents	Pertuzumab (Perjeta), tucatinib (Tukysa), neratinib (Nerlynx), lapatinib (Tykerb)
Drugs to treat hormone receptor–positive breast cancer	Abemaciclib (Verzenio), alpelisib (Piqray)
Immuno-oncology	Pembrolizumab (Keytruda)
Infections	*Clostridium difficile* colitis
Antibiotic use	Most antibiotics can cause diarrhea.
Laxative use	Most laxatives can cause loose stools.

while she still has some loose stools, they only happen every few days and she feels like she can predict when they are coming. So she's back to golfing and reported it felt great to get back to something she loves doing.

Bowel trouble is no fun, but your doctor will continue to work to find a combination of medications to minimize your discomfort. It's the constant dialog with your medical team that will make the difference. Tell your medical team about the frequency and consistency of your bowel movements, and then compare these to your normal baseline. If your stools are very loose or watery for more than a day, call the clinic. While it may feel embarrassing to call the clinic with bowel issues, we are harder to shock than new mothers in that we talk about poop and vomit all day long.

Treating Diarrhea

Your doctor will determine what she thinks is the underlying cause of your diarrhea, which will help her strategize the best approach to treating it. In some cases the fix is straightforward. For example, if you've taken too many laxatives, that's simple to reverse. Sometimes, when the cause is the cancer treatments, the fix is less straightforward. Your doctor may continue your cancer treatment as planned and simply try to treat the symptoms alone. If this is not effective, your doctor may adjust the doses of cancer therapies to address the diarrhea. Patients sometimes worry about reporting how much diarrhea they are experiencing because they may be concerned that their doctor may decrease or modify their treatments. It's important to let your team know about your symptoms because diarrhea can lead to dehydration and a host of other problems.

Some people may benefit from IV fluids administered at times when diarrhea is worst. One of the healthiest patients Jenn has ever treated is Lena, a 32-year-old mother of three. She was running several marathons a year and taking daily spin classes when she was diagnosed with an early-stage HER2-positive breast cancer. Her neoadjuvant chemotherapy regimen included pertuzumab, which is a HER2 treatment that can cause diarrhea in some people. Lena reported some loose stools after her first infusion, but insisted things were under control. We tried several antidiarrheal medications for her second cycle. The next week Jenn could tell from the lab work that Lena was probably having a lot more diarrhea than she admitted to, and Jenn asked her to come into the infusion unit for a couple of days of IV fluids.

After her third cycle of chemo, she was hospitalized with severe diarrhea and dehydration. Jenn then dropped the pertuzumab, and Lena sailed through her remaining cycles of chemo with no bowel issues. She had been really scared to change anything in the planned chemo regimen, but the toxicity of the pertuzumab for her was really significant despite our best attempts to control the diarrhea. In the end, she had a pathologic complete response to the therapy, meaning no disease left in the breast after neoadjuvant treatment, and this was even without all of her cycles of pertuzumab. Most times, we are able to control diarrhea with medications, but it may be helpful to know that your doctors can also adjust the cancer treatments if needed.

There are three primary drugs that doctors use to treat diarrhea: loperamide (Imodium), diphenoxylate and atropine (Lomotil), and tincture of opium.

Loperamide (Imodium)

This is the first line of defense against diarrhea. It's an opioid that doesn't get absorbed into the central nervous system but instead binds with opioid receptors in the intestines and causes the GI tract to slow down. It is available over the counter and comes in 2-milligram tablets or capsules. You can safely take a starting dose of two tablets, followed by one tablet every six hours for diarrhea. Sometimes for chemotherapy-induced diarrhea, we ask patients to take one tablet every hour until the diarrhea stops. Generally it's not recommended to take more than eight tablets (16 milligrams) a day. If you find that you need to take more or if the diarrhea lasts for more than half a day despite taking hourly loperamide, you need to call your doctor.

Diphenoxylate and Atropine (Lomotil)

If loperamide doesn't have a positive effect, then the next drug that we often try is called Lomotil, which is a combination of diphenoxylate and atropine. Diphenoxylate is another opioid-like drug. Unlike loperamide, this drug can be absorbed into the central nervous system and can cause euphoria, but it doesn't control pain very well. Like loperamide, it works primarily in the intestinal tract to slow peristalsis. Manufacturers have combined it with atropine, which can cause tachycardia (a fast heart rate) if taken in high doses. But it can often have a positive antidiarrheal effect where other drugs have failed.

Tincture of Opium

This is usually the next-most aggressive drug we can try if others aren't working. Tincture of opium is also called laudanum or deodorized tincture of opium. It is a very strong antidiarrheal, so strong in fact that it is administered in drops. Doctors usually prescribe this drug when Imodium or Lomotil are ineffective.

CHAPTER ELEVEN

Minimizing Pain

Pain is one of the symptoms that palliative care specialists and oncologists take the most seriously. Not everyone who has cancer gets pain, but if you do have pain, we want it to be well controlled. Living with pain is exhausting. You can't be yourself and do the things you love to do if you are constantly thinking about pain. And yet, this is the one area where patients seem to struggle the most to communicate how they feel. So many times I (Vicki) hear patients say, "Well, it hurts so much that I can't walk, but I don't want to take anything." Or they say, "I can't sleep at night because of the pain, but if I take something, won't I become an addict?"

You should never expect to live with unmanaged pain, and if your pain is interfering with your daily life, keeping you in your bed or on your couch, or even keeping you from spending time with your family, you need help.

The experience of pain is intensely personal, something that can make you feel vulnerable and even anxious about the future, and I understand that some people feel uncomfortable talking about it. Many times patients will tell an oncologist—even one they really like and trust—that they have no real problems with pain. Then, on the same day, they come to an appointment with me or with someone in palliative care, and the first subject they want to discuss is how they can't sleep because of the pain or how the medication offered so far isn't helping. When I ask why they didn't bring this up with the oncologist, the answers are often similar:

"I thought there was supposed to be pain."

"I don't want him to think I'm weak or can't take the chemotherapy."

"What if the cancer is getting worse? I don't want her to stop the chemotherapy."

You should never expect to have poorly controlled pain just because you have cancer, and nobody will think you are weak. While new or increasing pain might be a sign that the cancer is advancing, it might be due to something else entirely. Your oncologist wants to help you manage pain, and most oncologists have training in pain management. But sometimes pain is tricky to manage, and it may require more than one medication or strategy. You have to continue to communicate your symptoms so that the doctor can figure out the right approach to treat not just the pain but the cancer itself.

If your doctor has prescribed a pain regimen that isn't working, you need speak up so that he or she can make adjustments or consult with a pain specialist like a palliative care clinician. Sometimes there is a little bit of fine-tuning of medications before we can find a solution that reduces pain, but when I meet with patients in the palliative care clinic, I am always very clear that we can reduce their pain.

Postoperative Pain

If you will undergo breast surgery, you can expect to experience postoperative pain that is usually transient in nature. It may last for a few days or a few weeks depending on the type of surgery. If that pain persists or worsens, you will want to talk to your team about it. They will want to make sure that you are healing appropriately. Sometimes women develop fluid in the surgical area called a seroma, and this may need to be drained. Rarely, women may develop an infection or bleeding in the surgical site, which can also cause pain.

While it is common to experience intermittent pangs of breast pain that occur even years after surgery, this pain is not usually persistent and does not typically require any pain medications. Women may notice this when the area is pushed on or during a breast exam. Other women describe chronic, fleeting pains in the breast or armpit that come on suddenly and resolve on their own. Patients are often reassured when I tell them that this is the experience of lots of women and does not usually mean anything worrisome about cancer recurrence. If your pain is persistent and getting worse over time, however, it is important to let your team know, so that you can be checked out.

Cancer-Related Pain

Women with metastatic breast cancer can experience pain as tumors grow or press on different tissues, bones, and nerves. We call this chronic cancer pain or cancer-related pain. This pain from cancer often improves as the tumor shrinks and responds to therapy. Sometimes the pain might not resolve completely even if the treatments are working well. The main focus of this chapter is to provide guidance on how to deal with chronic cancer pain.

Describing the Intensity of Pain

At every visit to the clinic, someone in your medical team should be asking you whether your pain is acceptable and whether pain is interfering with your normal life. You will be asked whether you have any new pain. This is called a pain assessment. If you do have pain, you will be asked to describe its intensity and qualities. Is it dull or sharp? Can you easily identify the location, or is the pain diffuse? Is it a shooting pain that seems to radiate from one point to another? Does it burn or ache? Is it intermittent or constant? Does it increase or decrease at certain times of day? Is it worse when you move or sit or stand in a certain way?

These questions help your team figure out why you may be experiencing pain and what might help you feel better. If you develop new areas of discomfort, your doctor needs to know about it. Even if you don't think that your pain is related to your cancer, you should still discuss it with your doctor. The sudden emergence of back pain or pain in your bones can alert your medical team to changes in your health. Also, some patients experience pain in areas that have nothing to do with their tumors.

Your doctor will ask you to rate your pain on a scale of 0 to 10 and might present you with a pain scale with numbers and faces on it (figure 11.1). This scale is confusing for many people, but doctors understand that pain is subjective, and your sensitivity to it will be affected by other factors, including your general health, your mood, and your level of fatigue. I typically explain it this way: it is unlikely that you will have 0 pain but more likely that we will be able to keep your cancer pain in the 1 to 2 range. The low end of the scale, 1 to 3, represents pain that you notice but that doesn't interfere with your life. With a pain level of 2, most patients can still read the paper or engross themselves in a movie.

You can ignore it enough to continue to do almost everything you want. Sometimes you may be tempted to treat this pain with over-the-counter analgesics like acetaminophen, ibuprofen, or aspirin. Please don't take these medicines without asking someone on your medical team. While your team may recommend these medications, there may be reasons your doctor wouldn't want you to treat pain with these types of medications, and there may be better solutions for you.

Moderate pain, between 4 and 6, represents pain that interferes with your daily activities. As part of my pain assessment, I always ask, "Is there anything that you want to do that you can't do because of the pain?" The answer to this question helps me to know how to best treat it. Sometimes patients are fine if they are sitting but then have pain when they get up to walk, while other patients have pain that worsens when they are lying in bed, making it difficult to get a good night's sleep. Moderate pain almost always requires treatment with an opioid pain medication, such as morphine or oxycodone. Some people have various reservations or concerns about taking opioids, but you will likely be starting at a low dose.

If your moderate pain is intermittent, meaning that it comes and goes, you might take an opioid as needed. However, if the pain is constant, your doctor might suggest that you take a short- or long-acting medication on a regular schedule. I am never worried about how much or what type of medication is needed to treat the pain as long as the patient has good pain control and few side effects from the medications.

Severe pain, anything above a 7, is serious and something your doctors will want to treat aggressively. In this situation, you might have a tough time doing anything but think about the pain. Some patients have told me that they have to hold perfectly still or they have to keep pacing to manage the pain. Your team needs to know about this kind of pain immediately. With the right treatments, even severe pain can be made better. Remember, our goal is to get the pain intensity down to that 1 to 2 range. We might not be able to eliminate your pain, but we can reduce it enough to improve your quality of life. Doctors often combine medications and treatments to reduce severe pain.

I met Sarah shortly after she was admitted to Mass General with a diagnosis of breast cancer. Breast cancers tend to metastasize (spread) to the bone, and Sarah was having terrible pain in her left hip from a

Wong-Baker FACES® Pain Rating Scale

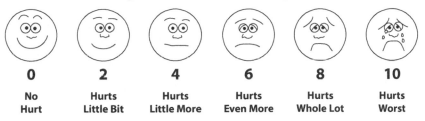

0	2	4	6	8	10
No Hurt	Hurts Little Bit	Hurts Little More	Hurts Even More	Hurts Whole Lot	Hurts Worst

Figure 11.1. Your doctor may use the Wong-Baker FACES® Pain Rating Scale during your cancer pain assessment. Used with permission from Wong-Baker FACES Foundation, retrieved August 19, 2016, http://www.WongBakerFACES.org.

bone metastasis. The pain was so bad that she couldn't walk, stand up to shower, or spend time with her family. In fact, she told me that she had to slide herself across the floor to get from one room to another and that her children were really frightened by this. In fact, she cried when she described her children's fears to me. And yet, when I asked her about taking medication for pain, she told me that she thought she should be tough enough to handle the pain, even though the scans revealed that she had a large tumor in the bones of her pelvis.

Before her diagnosis, Sarah had been incredibly active and fit. She played competitively in a women's hockey league two to three times a week. Her children and husband also played hockey. "This is what we do together," she told me. "This is important to me. I want to play hockey again."

I started her on the short-acting opioid oxycodone every three hours and ibuprofen every eight hours. This improved her pain in the short term so that she could function more normally. In addition, she started radiation to reduce the pain in her hip. I also started her on a low dose of long-acting oxycodone, which is a pain medication that lasts eight to twelve hours. Most patients with cancer pain need a combination of long- and short-acting pain medications if they have steady pain in addition to acute pain with some activity.

With these medications, Sarah had her pain down to a 2 out of 10. After radiation and some physical therapy, she was able to go back to playing hockey, and she felt like herself again.

Treatments for Pain

Actively engage your medical team about the symptoms of pain and how treatments are working. You can copy table 11.1 and use it to track your symptoms and the effectiveness of any treatments you receive. This will help your medical team assess your dosage and recommend alternatives if your current medication isn't working or has too many side effects.

Nonopioid Pain Relievers

Ibuprofen and naproxen are both nonsteroidal anti-inflammatory drugs, commonly called NSAIDs. These medications can be incredibly helpful in treating any pain caused by inflammation, including bone pain. In truth, most types of pain have some inflammatory component, which is why NSAIDs are so often prescribed. You do need to be careful, though. These medications can cause irritation in the stomach and even lead to an ulcer, so it's important to take them with some food. Or your doctor may also recommend a medication that reduces the stomach's production of acid, such as omeprazole or another proton pump inhibitor. Even with these additional drugs, though, you can still develop an ulcer. NSAIDs can also affect the kidneys and how they function, so they need to be used very cautiously in patients with kidney problems. Your doctor will want you to monitor for any signs of bleeding while taking an NSAID.

Your clinician will be also looking for other nonopioid treatment for your pain. Acetaminophen can be helpful as an extra medication to treat pain. Other medications, including gabapentin or tricyclic antidepressants (amitriptyline or nortriptyline), can be helpful in the treatment for neuropathic (nerve) pain. Any of these can be prescribed before opioids or in conjunction with opioids.

For many patients with early-stage cancer who have just had breast surgery, nonopioid pain relievers may be enough to treat the pain experienced from the surgery. This is especially true when recovering from a lumpectomy. If you've had a mastectomy or if several lymph nodes have been removed from your armpit, you may benefit from a few days of a short-acting opioid. Surgeons sometimes recommend a couple of weeks of gabapentin to help with postoperative nerve pain.

Table 11.1. Tracking pain and pain management at home

Date and time	Pain location and description	Pain intensity (0–10)	Medication taken and dosage	Effect at one hour: Pain intensity (0–10)	Nonpharmacologic strategies used (e.g., ice, heating pad, relaxation, distraction)

Short-Acting Opioids

Most patients will require the addition of a short-acting opioid pain medication like morphine or oxycodone to effectively manage cancer-related pain. These medications bind with opioid receptors in areas of the body, including the brain and spinal cord, and reduce your perception of pain. Most short-acting opioids take about an hour to reach peak effect and last somewhere between two and four hours, depending on the intensity of the pain.

If you have intermittent pain or pain associated with a particular activity, you know that the pain might start slowly and peak for a time before it starts to fade. Your doctor may tell you to take a short-acting opioid when the pain starts, so that it increases in effectiveness as the pain increases and then fades roughly when the pain itself will fade. It may be tempting to wait as long as possible before taking the pill, thinking that you should tough it out. But when you do that, you risk doing what we call "overshooting the pain." That means that the opioid takes full effect after the pain has gone away, and that might leave you feeling groggy when you want to be more alert.

One caution about using short-acting opioids: it is best to use preparations that do not contain acetaminophen as a combination product. For example, Percocet contains both oxycodone and acetaminophen, and Vicodin contains both hydrocodone and acetaminophen. These aren't good choices if you need to take an opioid every three hours to manage your pain because it is not safe to take acetaminophen that frequently. Doctors usually recommend dosing acetaminophen separately from the short-acting opioid.

Long-Acting Opioids

If you find yourself taking a short-acting opioid at regular intervals throughout the day, your doctor may suggest that you switch to a long-acting opioid (table 11.2), which is a similar medication but the effects last for many more hours. Some opioids come in both a short-acting and a long-acting form. Oxycodone and morphine both have long-acting pills that last eight to twelve hours. These are also known as controlled-release or extended-release preparations (sometimes written out as CR or ER in prescriptions). Although manufacturers suggest taking a new dose every twelve hours, we have found that it is not uncommon for the pain relief to fall short of the full twelve hours, and you may need to take a new dose after eight. Fentanyl comes in a patch that goes on the skin and typically lasts 72 hours. Methadone is another opioid that can be used as a long-acting medication, but it works a bit differently and requires special precautions, so I will describe it in a separate section.

Most often in the outpatient setting we start with medications taken by mouth or patches that are placed on the skin. Many clinicians like to start with oral medications if possible, because it is easier to adjust the dosage as needed. Your doctor may suggest a fentanyl patch if you are having nausea and can't reliably keep down pills or because it is just easier for you to remember to put a patch on every three days rather than taking a pill two or three times per day.

The downside of using a patch is that it can take 12 to 24 hours to fully kick in whenever you change the dose. The patch works by seeping into the thin layer of fatty tissue beneath the skin. Patients can struggle to find the right dose if they have lost a great deal of weight during their illness.

Methadone for Pain

Methadone is a long-acting opioid that you may have heard about as a treatment for heroin addiction. But what you might not know is that it is also an extremely effective, inexpensive, high-potency pain medication sometimes prescribed to treat cancer pain. It may be especially helpful for pain from nerve irritation, the kind that feels like shooting or burning pain.

Table 11.2. Equivalent intravenous (IV) to oral dosing for opioids

Opioid	IV	Oral dose
Oxycodone	n/a	20 mg
Morphine	10 mg	30 mg
Hydromorphone	1.5 mg	7.5 mg

Methadone is a terrific opioid for severe pain, but it can be very tricky to administer, so you want to make sure that your clinicians have experience prescribing it. Unlike other opioids, methadone takes three to five days to reach peak effect. You and your clinician will need to devise a plan to manage your pain aggressively for those first three days. Your doctor may give you additional short-acting opioids to take in these first few days, or she may recommend taking some steroids during this period of time. After three days, your doctor can safely increase the methadone.

You never want to overshoot the dose of methadone because it can be unsafe at high levels. I tell patients to be aware of how they feel during those first two days of using methadone. The crazy thing is this: If you feel great on day one or day two, we may have given you too much. That's why you will need to be communicating with your medical team frequently if you start a course of methadone.

Remember to take the methadone exactly as prescribed. Never increase your use of methadone without guidance from your clinical team.

Timing Pain Medications

It's sometimes tricky to figure out how to time pain medications; people are sometimes tempted to hold off as long as they can before taking anything for relief. When Dave explains the timing of these medications, he sometimes draws a graph on a piece of paper that illustrates the normal ebb and flow of cancer pain through a typical day (figure 11.2). There are often normal variations in pain caused by physical movement or other factors, and these are sometimes predictable. The shading on the next graph shows how the pain medication starts and builds slowly to full effect and then wears off (figure 11.3). You can see how the pain medication taken was more than was needed in two out of the four spikes. When you wait to take medication, sometimes the short-acting medication is reaching peak effect when the pain is less severe. We refer to this as "overshooting the pain" and in that case people experience drowsiness (sedation). It's important to remember that short-acting medications last just three to four hours, and patients can experience erratic pain control.

Long-Acting Plus Short-Acting Medication

Patients with chronic cancer pain will usually need both a long- and a short-acting opioid. The long-acting opioid treats the baseline pain and provides a constant level of pain relief. It is much more effective because

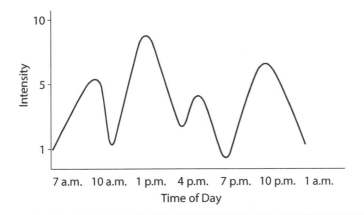

Figure 11.2. Pain without opioids

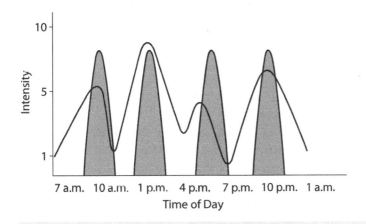

Figure 11.3. Pain with short-acting opioids; shaded areas indicate pain relief

it doesn't cause the peaks and valleys that you get with short-acting pain meds alone. If you just take short-acting pills in succession, you will have peak times when you feel drowsy, and then, as the pill wears off, you will be in a valley with more intense pain until you take the next dose. A long-acting medication will give you moderate pain control all the time, and then you can take an additional short-acting dose when the pain breaks through. This so-called breakthrough pain can happen two or three times per day. If it happens more often than that, we typically use this as a cue to increase the long-acting medication.

One of my patients was experiencing significant back and hip pain from bony metastases at the time of her diagnosis with metastatic breast cancer. She experienced near constant pain to the point where she couldn't leave her house. When the pain would spike, Loretta would take a short-acting opioid. She said that it offered relief but also made her drowsy and feel "out of it." If she took a pill just before people came to visit her, she would often have to excuse herself to take a nap. She was starting to feel kind of isolated. I suggested a long-acting opioid that could give her better pain control throughout the day.

Loretta's daughter, who is a nurse, worried that adding another opioid would make the drowsiness worse. I explained that a long-acting opioid could provide better pain control with less sedation. Loretta decided to try a long-acting morphine preparation twice a day. When I called to touch base a few days later, Loretta said she couldn't believe how much better she felt. She was able to play bridge with her friends and enjoy time with her grandchildren without being in severe pain and without dozing off.

I always remind people that in almost every case we can treat pain to bring it down to an acceptable level. Long-acting pain medications can be an important tool in the tool box.

When we start a long-acting opioid, as in figure 11.4, patients experience a much more consistent treatment of their pain. We can still use short-acting opioids for any pain not adequately controlled by the long-acting medication. In general after we start a long-acting opioid, most patients will need the short-acting medication just two to three times per day, as you can see in figure 11.5.

Being Proactive About Pain

It's worth noting again that a common mistake patients make is letting the pain get ahead of them. It's tempting to think that you can handle the pain and take care of it later. Patients sometimes tell me that they didn't call the clinic when their pain became disruptive because they didn't want to bother anyone, or they thought they could wait it out until the next medical visit. The trouble is that your pain can escalate over a couple of days, and then it becomes harder to treat. Go ahead and call the clinic if your pain is getting worse. Someone on your team can help you.

If you are taking a short-acting opioid, I suggest that my patients take

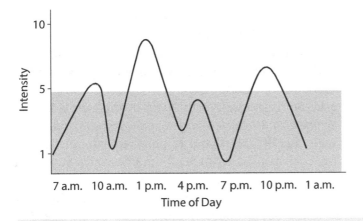

Figure 11.4. Pain with long-acting opioids; shaded area indicates pain relief

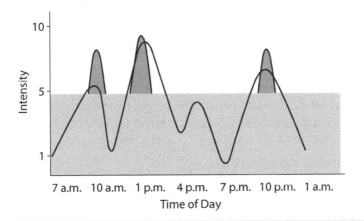

Figure 11.5. Pain with short- and long-acting opioids; lighter shading indicates pain relief from long-acting medications; darker shading indicates pain relief from short-acting medications

these medications every three to four hours as needed to keep the pain at an acceptable level so they can do the activities that matter to them. Remember that short-acting opioids are meant to be taken on an as-needed basis. If you don't have bothersome pain, you don't need to take them on a regular basis.

If you are taking a long-acting opioid, you want to avoid skipping doses. Sometimes people are tempted to skip doses of the long-acting opioid if they aren't in pain, but it's the medication that is often controlling the underlying pain. If you skip a dose, the pain can get ahead of you. Devise a system so you don't forget a dose, because your overall pain control will be worse if you skip doses. Sometimes people set their phone to alert when they are due for a dose. Or they take it with other scheduled medications.

Make sure to track your responses to the pain medication you have been given. You may want to do this in writing or bring someone with you to clinic visits who can talk about your response to pain medication and how it's working. Your medical team wants to know how your pain medications affect you. If the doses make you feel sedated and sleepy when you want to be more active and engaged with your family, your doctor can help you find a better dose for those times of the day. The goal is to have you feeling alert but with good pain control. Sometimes pain can be difficult to manage, and you may need to decide whether you would prefer to have a little more pain but be more alert or have a little less pain and be more sleepy.

Sarah, whom I mentioned earlier, had good pain control with her oral regimen but experienced sedation. We added a low dose of methylpheni- date (a stimulant that is sometimes used to treat attention deficit disor- der and can also be helpful for cancer-related fatigue) each morning and at noon, and she was able to have good pain control and still be alert.

Side Effects and Other Common Concerns

Opioids are wonderfully helpful in treating cancer pain, but they can have some side effects that we need to be aware of and manage. These include constipation, nausea, and grogginess. Not everyone experiences all of the side effects. In fact, many of my patients start opioids and don't experience any except for constipation, which is the most persistent side effect and the main side effect you want to be aware of when starting to take an opioid (for a discussion of the laxatives doctors usually prescribe alongside opioids, see chapter 10).

While you may feel groggy or experience some nausea during the first few days of taking an opioid, these feelings should subside within a few days, or a week at most. In those first few days after starting an opioid, I suggest that patients have a medication available to take if they feel any nausea (see chapter 9).

Some patients worry about their breathing slowing down on opioids.

Opioids are highly unlikely to cause respiratory depression if they are taken as prescribed. Patients who are taking large doses of other sedating medications, such as lorazepam, and also patients with renal failure, pulmonary issues, or sleep apnea should discuss appropriate dosing with their clinician. Pain can be effectively and safely treated with opioids. You just need to work with your care team to find what works best for you. It's normal to be concerned that you may need multiple medications or treatments to reduce your pain.

Many patients have asked me whether they will become an addict because they are taking medications sometimes associated with addiction or abuse. Others fear that the medications won't make their life normal, or that they will lose effectiveness over time. Let's take these one by one.

Am I Going to Become Addicted?

It's highly unlikely that you will become addicted to your pain medication. In the vast majority of cases, patients with cancer can take opioids effectively just as they are prescribed. If you are taking opioids after breast surgery, you will be given enough medication to help you in the recovery period. Very rarely are people taking opioids beyond a few weeks after surgery.

Those patients taking opioids to treat pain from advanced cancer can—in most cases—take these medications safely as prescribed as well. These opioids are powerful medications, but the key to avoiding issues related to addiction is to take the medications only as prescribed and to take pain medications for pain only. If you are having anxiety, we should treat it with a medication for anxiety, not a pain medication. Additionally, pain medications help you engage more fully in life. Good pain control means that you can do what you want to do, unlike people with addiction issues, who use opioids to withdraw from life.

Can I Drive While Taking Opioids?

The short answer is no. You should not drive while taking opioids. The long answer is that people who are on a stable dose of long-acting opioids for well-established pain might be able to drive without feeling impaired. But this has never been proven. From a legal standpoint, I tell patients that if you do choose to drive and if you cause an accident or injure someone, you may have no legal defense against the accusation that you were impaired.

Will Pain Medicine Make My Life Normal?

The goal of pain medication is to reduce the discomfort that would prevent you from living as fully as you can. Cancer changes your life, and some activities that you used to do may not be possible, but most patients can do a great deal of what they loved before. The key is to reframe your expectations. One of my patients is an avid runner. She loved the challenge of setting personal-best times to beat in each race. When her pain from bony metastases worsened, she was not able to run. After we found a regimen that worked for her, she was able to do some jogging, which felt great. She wasn't training the way she used to and didn't feel up for running a race, but she was so glad to be active again and decided to try trail running and running along the beach.

What If They Stop Working?

Another worry that patients have is that pain medications will lose their effectiveness over time. Sometimes patients ask if they should hold off on starting an opioid because they worry that they should save these medications for when they get sicker and really need it. It is true that bodies get more efficient at processing these medications over time, which is called tolerance. Your medical team will know how to compensate to find reasonable pain control. All opioids have different potencies (e.g., 20 mg of oxycodone is equivalent to 7.5 mg of oral hydromorphone), and if we find that one opioid isn't working as well as it needs to, you can switch to another. I have had patients who required hundreds of milligrams of opioids per day over the course of several years in order to function. Rest assured your doctor can figure something out. He or she can also refer you to a pain specialist, such as a palliative care clinician. We have lots of expertise in managing complex pain syndromes.

Can I Just Stop Taking Them?

If you are taking opioids for just a few days after surgery, you can stop whenever you want. However, if you are taking these medications long term for cancer-related pain, you should ask your team for guidance on when you might come off them. If your pain decreases dramatically, your doctor can reduce the dosage. Do not stop taking opioids abruptly, though, because you can have rebound pain that is difficult to get under control, and it's possible to have a pain crisis if you stop taking your pain medication suddenly.

Other Strategies for Serious Pain

If you have a sudden, severe onset of pain, your doctor might consider giving pain medication through an IV infusion. Medication delivered in this way typically reaches peak effect in 15 minutes. You will probably have to be in a hospital setting to receive IV pain medication, but this allows your clinician to quickly figure out how much medication you need and then convert this dosage to an oral regimen you can use at home.

Some patients who need more constant access to IV pain medication can use a patient-controlled analgesia (PCA) pump that is attached to an IV line. This allows patients to give themselves pain relief as needed in a hospital setting. You can just press a button, and the machine will give you a dose of pain medication. Your doctor might suggest this if you are having trouble with oral medications or if your stomach is having trouble absorbing the medication.

These PCA pumps can be portable enough for patients to take home if necessary. Patients will need to have a longer-term IV, called a PICC line or a port, that the medication infuses into, and they will have a small pump for the pain medication to carry with them at all times. It usually fits into a fanny pack.

Other patients may benefit from a form of opioid delivery called an intrathecal pump. It delivers pain medication directly to the spinal cord, allowing doctors to prescribe a much lower dose. It does require a trial of the approach to make sure it will work for the patient's particular kind of pain and then a small surgery to implant the pump into the abdomen. It is a great option for certain patients.

Treatments for Localized Pain

When doctors ask patients to describe the pain associated with cancer, they will always ask about location. Is the pain in a defined area, or does it seem to be located inside a bone? Sometimes tumors cause serious pain in a small, well-defined area. If so, your medical team may look to treat that area rather than giving opioids alone.

Palliative Radiation

While radiation is usually given to kill cancer cells and shrink tumors, it has the side benefit of reducing the pain caused by these tumors. This can be particularly effective if the cancer has metastasized inside a bone.

Rather than using radiation to completely remove the tumor, which may not be possible, the treatments can contain it and dramatically reduce the pain it causes. One of my patients was struggling with pain from a tumor in her hip. After radiation, her pain decreased dramatically.

Sometimes a breast or chest-wall mass can grow and even break through the skin, causing pain, ulceration, discharge, and bleeding. If cancer treatments are not working to control this, sometimes palliative radiation can help control the pain and bleeding.

Nerve Blocks

Another strategy to deal with pain not well controlled by medication is something called a nerve block. An anesthesiologist or pain specialist can inject a substance into or around a nerve to numb it and prevent it from sending pain sensations to the brain. This helps control pain contained in one specific area of the body or limit the amount of opioids needed in general.

CHAPTER TWELVE

Should I Worry about Shortness of Breath?

Sometimes breast cancer patients report a sense that they are a little more winded than usual, and they wonder if that's a result of the cancer or cancer treatment. It can be disconcerting to get to the top of the stairs and have to take a break to catch your breath. There are several benign reasons why your breathing may change while in treatment, but a few are more serious.

If you find yourself winded going up the stairs or if you can't engage in normal levels of activity without a tightness in your chest or feeling the need to rest to catch your breath, you want to talk to your medical team who will help figure out what might be going on. There are a lot of strategies your doctor can use to help you breathe easier. Oncologists know that shortness of breath is a side effect that can reduce your appetite and make you less mobile and more isolated. It can also cause anxiety or even a panic attack.

The first thing that people worry about is whether they are taking in enough oxygen. But in most cases your lungs are fine, and your body is getting enough oxygen. The feeling of breathlessness is actually the feeling that your body is working harder to get air in and out of the lungs. Your diaphragm and chest muscles are working harder to expand and collapse to push the air in and out, and that is what causes the feeling of breathlessness.

Remember that every time you go to the clinic, the medical assistants are taking your vital signs, and that includes measuring your respiratory rate and the oxygen level in your blood. When patients come into the clinic complaining of shortness of breath, we take those same vital signs, and in many cases their oxygen level is fine. Then we know that it's the sensation of working harder to breathe that is the issue.

There are many reasons why a person with any stage of breast cancer may experience breathlessness:

- If you have not been moving or exercising much, you may be deconditioned and feel out of breath while walking up the stairs.

- In rare cases, chemotherapy and other cancer treatments can cause a type of inflammation called interstitial pneumonitis, which is swelling in the lining of your lungs, making it difficult to take a full breath. There are also some treatments like trastuzumab that can impact the pumping function of your heart, which can lead to fluid buildup in the lungs and subsequent shortness of breath.

- You could have a blood clot that reduces blood flow to the heart or lungs. Many blood clots are "silent," meaning they don't cause any symptoms, but some may cause shortness of breath, chest pain, or lightheadedness, depending on the extent and location of the clot.

- You may have low blood counts, meaning there aren't enough red blood cells to carry oxygen to your cells, making you feel that you need to breathe harder even though your lungs are working fine.

- Anxiety or panic can also make you feel short of breath.

If you have advanced breast cancer, there are additional reasons why you may feel short of breath:

- Your abdomen may be filling up with fluid (ascites), and it's harder for you to contract and flatten your diaphragm and thus have your lungs fill up with air.

- The space around your lungs may be filling up with fluid (pleural effusion), making it more difficult to move your diaphragm or for your lungs to expand with air.

- The cancer may have spread to your lungs, and a tumor or spray of small tumors along the lining of your lungs (pleura) may be making it hard for your lungs to expand.

- The cancer may be spreading along the alveoli, the building blocks of the lungs, making it harder for your lungs to expand. This is known as lymphangitic spread or carcinomatosis.

- You may have pneumonia caused by the cancer blocking one of the bronchi (air passages leading from the trachea to the lungs).

- Fluid may be building up along the lining of your heart (pericardium), making it more difficult for the heart to move blood through your lungs and making them boggy like a sponge.

Although any one of these causes will interfere with the ease of breathing, none of them usually affect your lungs' ability to take in oxygen, except in severe cases.

Diagnosing the Cause

Your medical team will work to figure out what might be causing your shortness of breath. Your doctor may order a chest CT to look for any fluid in the lungs or small tumors. Sometimes you may need an additional test, such as a CT angiogram, also called a pulmonary embolism protocol CT, which uses an IV contrast to check for blood clots in the arteries that feed the lungs. In some cases your doctor may order an echocardiogram, which is an ultrasound that shows how the heart is working. The heart muscle can be damaged by cancer or by cancer therapy, or it may be surrounded by fluid from the cancer, and an echocardiogram is the best way to see whether that has happened.

The results of these tests will give your doctor some idea of how to treat the underlying cause (table 12.1). That might mean draining any accumulating fluid, treating pneumonia, or giving a blood transfusion for low blood counts. The goal of your medical team is to make you comfortable and reduce your anxiety even if the underlying cause of breathing troubles can't be treated. Here we'll cover some of the treatable causes.

Deconditioning

After you have been in treatment for a while, you may feel tired and avoid some of the activities that you have previously enjoyed. It's a good idea to maintain some level of activity when you are feeling strongest, such as getting out of the house to take a short walk. Without regular walks or movement, your muscles will begin to weaken, and then you are more likely to feel winded when you do move, even though your lungs are working just fine.

I (Jenn) first met Dora when she was admitted to the hospital with a hip fracture and was found to have hormone receptor–positive metastatic breast cancer. She started on hormonal therapy for the cancer and had

Table 12.1. Causes and treatment of shortness of breath

Causes	Treatment[1]
Fluid around the lungs (pleural effusion)	Drainage of the fluid with a catheter or chest tube
Inflammation in the lung (pneumonitis)	Steroids
Heart failure	Diuretics
Blood clot (pulmonary embolus)	Blood thinners
Fluid in the abdomen (ascites)	Drainage of fluid
Cancer in the lung (in the lining of the lung, in the lymphatic channels in the lung, or within the lung and airways)	Cancer therapy, oxygen, opioids
Anemia (low red blood cells)	Blood transfusion
Pneumonia	Antibiotics
Deconditioning (being out of shape)	Physical therapy

[1]After treating any reversible causes, opioids can be used to ease the feeling of shortness of breath.

surgery on her hip. Then she spent some time in a rehabilitation facility before returning home. During our first appointment in the clinic, Dora was surrounded by a half dozen family members, all of whom were worried about how weak she had become. Dora's main concern was feeling breathless when she walked around for more than a few minutes. Her oxygen levels were normal, and a CT scan of her chest did not show signs of a clot or progressive cancer.

When we met again, Dora admitted that she wasn't very active anymore. Her loving, doting family would not allow her to do anything for herself because they said they worried about her falling again. As a result, Dora said she ended up spending most of the day on the couch watching television. "Maybe I'm just out of shape," she said.

Realizing the detriment to her health, her family agreed to let her do more things on her own. Within a few months, Dora was taking walks in the morning with her husband and in the evening with her kids. She said she felt stronger overall and had stopped being bothered by the feeling of breathlessness. Even moderate regular exercise, like Dora was getting, can increase lung capacity.

Pneumonitis

Cancer treatments and radiation can sometimes cause a reaction called pneumonitis. It sounds scary, but it simply means that white blood cells have infiltrated the lungs and attached to the lining of the alveoli. Doctors treat this with steroids. If there was a specific drug that caused the pneumonitis, usually your doctor will discontinue use of the drug, too.

Pneumonitis is a rare side effect of paclitaxel, a chemotherapy agent that can be used to treat both early-stage and advanced breast cancer. I was treating Sandy, an active nurse with an early-stage breast cancer, with paclitaxel when she called to say she was having difficulty climbing the stairs at work. She said, "I feel like I just ran one of my 5Ks after climbing two flights of stairs." Because she had continued to work during treatment, she wondered if the chemotherapy was just catching up with her. We brought her in for a visit and decided to check a CT of her chest, which showed pneumonitis. I started her on steroids, and she felt much better, and we did not give her the final cycle of paclitaxel.

Sandy worried about not completing all of her cycles of chemotherapy. This is a common and understandable concern, but the risk of worsening lung damage from more treatment far outweighs the benefits of continuing. She started on her hormonal therapy with tamoxifen and is feeling great years later with no permanent signs of lung damage.

At around the same time, I started to treat Ling, also a very active woman in her sixties, for metastatic HER2-positive breast cancer. She did great with her first few weeks of paclitaxel, trastuzumab, and pertuzumab, but after about six weeks she developed a persistent cough and shortness of breath even when resting. A CT scan showed pneumonitis. After stopping paclitaxel and starting on steroids, Ling's cough resolved. Years later, her metastatic cancer remains stable on trastuzumab and pertuzumab, and she continues to feel great, walking around her neighborhood for an hour each morning.

Blood Clot

Blood clots are common among cancer patients because cancer makes your blood more prone to clotting (see chapter 15). Additionally, there are some treatments like tamoxifen that carry a small risk of causing clots. Blood clots typically form along the lining of the veins of the legs and pelvis. They then break off and can go to your lungs. Often, they are silent and we pick them up on routine CT scans. But sometimes they can cause acute chest pain and shortness of breath.

We usually treat patients who have blood clots with blood thinners like enoxaparin. Unfortunately, these medications are given by subcutaneous injection (under the skin), which are inconvenient and can be uncomfortable for some people. Patients have to give themselves these injections once or twice per day, depending upon the drug and the reason for taking it. However, there are oral drugs, such as apixaban (Eliquis), that work to thin the blood, and you can ask your doctor if this is an option for you.

Anemia

When patients are severely anemic, they can feel short of breath, particularly when they move around. The red blood cells carry oxygen to our tissues, and if we don't have enough red blood cells circulating, our muscles don't get enough oxygen. At rest, we have more than enough red blood cells to carry oxygen. But when we exercise or just have a brief episode of extreme exertion like running up a flight of stairs, our muscles, heart, and brain require much more oxygen. If we don't have enough reserve, we feel short of breath. If you report shortness of breath, your oncology team may order a blood draw to check your red blood cell count, or hematocrit (see chapter 5). Typically your hematocrit needs to fall well under 30 before you may start to feel short of breath. Normally, a person's hematocrit runs about 40. If your doctor thinks that your shortness of breath is due to a low red blood count, she might speak with you about whether you might benefit from a transfusion.

Fluid Buildup

As cancer advances, you might have tumors spreading to the lungs and causing a buildup of fluid in the pleural cavity, meaning in the space between the lungs and the thin membrane around the lungs. When fluid accumulates in that space, it prevents your lungs from expanding enough for you to take a full breath.

That's what happened with Sheila, a 58-year-old woman with breast cancer that had spread to her bones and to the lining of her lungs. She was initially on paclitaxel, a chemotherapy drug that we gave her once a week. Normally, she felt great on chemo, except for transient numbness and tingling in her hands and feet for a few days after her treatments—a normal side effect for this drug.

Gradually, Sheila noticed that she was short of breath after walking up stairs. When she talked to her doctor, he ordered a chest CT, and it showed more thickening of the pleura, which is the thin membrane around the lungs. This indicated that fluid was accumulating between her chest wall and her lungs, which sounds frightening, but we can drain that fluid. Her doctor ordered a thoracentesis. This is a procedure in which the radiologist numbs an area of skin on your back and puts a needle directly into the space where we see a pocket of fluid to drain it away. In Sheila's case, the radiologist removed a liter of fluid that she then sent to the lab to check it for cancer cells. After several days the radiologist told Sheila that she did have cancer cells in that fluid, meaning the cancer was spreading.

Her doctor switched her to a new chemotherapy drug called capecitabine, which is a pill rather than an infusion. After several weeks, Sheila noticed that she had more energy and wasn't getting short of breath as easily. When her doctor did another CT scan, he found that the fluid had disappeared, and she did quite well on this new regimen for many months.

If the fluid is continuously building up, you can undergo repeat thoracenteses to remove the fluid. Your doctor may suggest putting a catheter in place so that you can drain the fluid yourself when you feel short of breath. This may sound a little extreme, but the tubes themselves are thin and flexible, and you can avoid coming to the hospital to have the fluid drained.

Another possible procedure is called a pleurodesis. For this, a doctor will inject a substance like talc through a chest tube. This substance will cause an inflammatory reaction between the lining of the lung and the chest cavity that essentially seals the lining to the chest wall so that fluid can't accumulate there. A pleurodesis can be quite painful and requires a hospitalization. Given this, catheters are often preferred to a pleurodesis to treat chronic buildup of fluid around the lung from cancer.

Supplemental Oxygen

If your blood oxygen levels drop below 90%, you might consider getting an oxygen tank to provide supplemental oxygen. Psychologically, it may be difficult to admit that you need extra oxygen, but it might make you feel better and more energetic. And the converse is true as well. If your oxygen saturation is at or above 90%, you might not need supplemental oxygen. Some people say that they feel much better when on oxygen, even though it's not raising their oxygen saturation that much. What might also be beneficial in this case is sitting in front of a fan, because it will give you the sensation of taking in more air.

Why Your Doctor Might Suggest Opioid Medications

In some cases your doctor will be able to partially treat the underlying cause of your breathing issues but not all of it. In these cases, your doctor will likely prescribe a low dose of an opioid medication to ease the sensation of being short of breath. Opioids work wonderfully to take that feeling away, and you won't necessarily need significant doses. You may feel that you don't want to take an opioid, even a low dose, if you aren't in any physical pain, but it can dramatically improve your quality of life if you are feeling short of breath.

My patient Sunita moved to Boston from Florida where she had just been diagnosed with a recurrence of her breast cancer. She was initially diagnosed with an early-stage breast cancer years ago, and the breast cancer had now spread into the lymphatic channels of her lungs, also known as lymphangitic carcinomatosis. This was causing extreme shortness of breath. Her husband said that she had recently been out playing tennis with her friends, but in the previous week she had to take a break from making their bed in the morning in order to catch her breath. We started her on chemotherapy, but I also recommended a low dose of morphine to help with the sensation of breathlessness.

Like many people, she was initially hesitant to take morphine because she did not have any pain and worried about addiction. I explained that opioids are very effective to treat shortness of breath and that these medications can be used safely when taken to treat specific symptoms. And if you've gone through decades of life without misusing substances like opioids, it's unlikely to become an issue now.

Ultimately, Sunita tried morphine and felt more at ease with breathing soon after. That weekend, she left a message with our team to let us know that she was able to go out to dinner with her son and grandchildren. After the chemotherapy started working and shrinking the tumor in her lungs, her breathing improved dramatically and she rarely needed the morphine. After a couple of months, she took a trip back to Florida and was able to keep a tennis date with her friends.

Treating the Anxiety

The other issue your doctor should be asking you about is anxiety. Working harder to breathe causes a lot of anxiety, and feeling anxious can also cause shortness of breath. You are not a wimp because you are feeling anxious about your breathing, and it's really important to treat both of these symptoms. We often suggest cognitive behavioral therapy (CBT), which can help you manage the anxiety associated with feeling short of breath.

CBT is a form of psychotherapy in which the patient works with a therapist (typically a psychologist) who looks at the interaction of thoughts and behaviors on feelings. In the case of anxiety from shortness of breath, the therapist will work with you to identify certain thoughts and behaviors that will help mitigate the feeling of anxiety. Cognitive behavioral therapists can help you develop relaxation strategies to reduce anxiety. This might include visualization, such as imagining being on a mountaintop with lots of air moving around you. They can also help you reframe the sensation of shortness of breath. Many people worry that these sensations are proof that the cancer is getting worse, and they worry that it can't be managed. In truth, there are many treatments that will help. The CBT clinician will help you work through these fears, and that alone will help you reduce your general anxiety.

There are other techniques you can use to ease the sense of breathlessness and the anxiety that accompanies it. This may include sitting in front of a fan or keeping car windows open while you drive, which helps make your body feel as though it's taking in more air. Sometimes, though, anxiety becomes so overwhelming that we need to treat it with medications. Benzodiazepines are wonderful anxiolytics (literally "breaking anxiety") that are quite effective for people with episodic panic attacks. Other medications that can help people feel better with severe anxiety include antidepressants such as citalopram or antipsychotics such as olanzapine.

Can I Die from Being Short of Breath?

Usually shortness of breath is not directly related to metastatic breast cancer filling up in your lungs and more often related to an increased sensation of shortness of breath because your work of breathing has increased. But it is possible to die of lung failure if there is a progression of metastatic cancer in the lungs that does not respond to cancer treatment. Patients with progressive metastases in the lungs often fear that they will not be able to breathe or feel as though they are choking for air. If this is your worry, you will want to talk to your medical team about the steps they can take to avoid this as the lungs become less efficient. They can effectively treat shortness of breath with medications and will continue to remove any accumulating fluid and give you supplemental oxygen. They can also continue to offer medications to control pain and anxiety, and these can make a huge difference.

In rare cases, some people may need a continuous infusion of opioids to help with breathlessness, and we can do that with what we call patient-controlled analgesia (PCA, discussed in chapter 11). It's a portable device that can directly infuse opioids—sometimes morphine or hydromorphone—at a set dose. The device has a second component, which is a button that allows patients to give themselves an extra dose of medication, called a bolus, if needed. You might be familiar with a PCA if you know someone who has used one while recovering from surgery. You may need to be admitted as an inpatient in the hospital for the medical team to set the appropriate level of opioids and make you as comfortable as possible before sending you home with a PCA.

CHAPTER THIRTEEN

What If I'm Gaining or Losing Weight?

Most people expect some weight loss with a cancer diagnosis. It's true that some cancer treatments can cause you to feel more tired and less like eating, but breast cancer treatments are different from other cancer treatments in that many patients notice weight gain while in treatment. If you were diagnosed with an early-stage breast cancer and are gaining weight over time, it's likely that there are many factors at play—a combination of aging and metabolism as well as caloric intake and inactivity. In this chapter, I (Jenn) talk about some strategies for maintaining a healthy weight during treatment.

Of course, not everyone gains weight in treatment. Some patients do undergo dramatic weight loss, and this can also cause stress. A significant change in appearance is an undeniable signal to loved ones that you are dealing with cancer and that your love of food and family meals and cooking has been replaced at least in part by medicines and chemotherapy infusions and side effects. Loss of appetite can be a side effect that causes a lot of tension in a household, and doctors are used to seeing families fight openly about why the patient isn't eating. It's completely normal to be concerned when a cancer patient doesn't feel like eating much. This situation can trigger worries that the cancer is advancing or that the patient is giving up in some way. But this isn't necessarily the case. In this chapter, I'll also talk about how patients and families can manage the basic act of taking in calories and all of the emotions that come with it.

Why Am I Gaining Weight?

A common theme in follow-up appointments with my patients, especially those who were diagnosed with an early-stage breast cancer, is weight gain and what to do about it. There are numerous reasons breast cancer patients gain weight. Some women enter menopause shortly after their diagnosis, or they undergo treatments such as chemotherapy that can trigger menopause, which can cause a metabolic shift in how the body stores fat. You may be less active while in treatment, and this can cause weight gain. Or you may be eating differently because of the stress of the diagnosis and treatment. Some people feel that hormonal therapies, such as tamoxifen and the aromatase inhibitors, are contributing to weight gain. These drugs are associated with both weight gain and weight loss, and while they may play some part, they are not usually the only drivers for weight gain over time.

As boring as it sounds, you will probably have to rely on some of the same techniques you've used in the past to maintain a healthy weight:

- Increasing your physical activity with a goal of 150 minutes of moderate to vigorous exercise every week

- Reducing your intake of processed foods in favor of whole foods with at least five servings of fruits and vegetables each day

- Limiting your consumption of alcohol to no more than one drink per day

The good news is that these are all lifestyle changes that you can control. Many of my patients feel empowered by this idea that they can commit to lifestyle changes that will improve the way they look and feel. They can't control how their bodies will respond to treatment, but they can decide to eat better and be more active, even if they need extra support. Women with a history of early-stage breast cancer who are overweight or obese are more likely to have a recurrence of breast cancer. That's why many women are motivated to maintain a healthy weight as part of their overall plan for wellness.

One of my patients had already gained 30 pounds in the years after having her four children. Then she gained another 20 pounds after being treated with chemotherapy for early-stage breast cancer. She met with my nurse practitioner to outline practical steps that would help her lose weight. Her husband was supportive and agreed that they would both commit to a healthy diet and a little bit of exercise. They researched easy, healthy recipes and cooked together. They took evening walks together at first, then eventually joined a gym. When I saw her in follow-up six months later, she had lost more than 40 pounds, and so had her husband.

Many people ask if there is a specific diet they should try or specific foods that they should avoid. Women often ask about low carb, vegan, or ketogenetic diets that they've heard may have anti-cancer properties.

Others ask about avoiding sugar because they've heard it feeds cancer cells. In general, there is no good research that points to a single diet or any specific food restrictions that will reduce the risk of breast cancer recurrence. I usually recommend a healthy, balanced diet with the general guidelines as noted earlier. If going low carb or vegan feels good and works for you, I am in full support. But you should choose a diet plan that fits with your lifestyle.

You don't need to go to extremes or choose a highly restrictive meal plan in order to maintain a healthy weight, but a healthy weight is one of the best things you can do for your overall health. You can ask your team if they can refer you to a dietician or a lifestyle medicine clinic that can help you make practical diet and activity changes. Established programs like Weight Watchers help people think about choosing foods that contribute to a lifestyle change rather than dieting. It helps to find a group of people with a common mission who are holding each other accountable. If going to a group is not for you, there are also numerous apps for smartphones that can help with weight loss. Many of them help you track the calories and nutritional content of foods, which takes some time and effort but can help with weight loss. Some of these apps are free, while others may charge a fee for extra support, such as a virtual coach.

If you are trying to increase your activity level, I suggest starting slowly and working up to more vigorous exercise over time. Several YMCAs in the country offer the Livestrong Program, a free 12-week group exercise program with a focus on health and well-being for patients with a history of cancer.

What If I'm Retaining Fluid?

Sometimes weight gain is a product of extra fluid in your body. If fluid builds up in the legs or other parts of the body, we call it edema, which means swelling. Some chemotherapies and the steroids we use around the time of treatment cause edema. Edema can also be caused by low protein in the blood. Or it can occur when the lymph system gets blocked with small tumors. Your doctor may recommend elevating your legs, compression stockings, and increasing the protein in your diet to help reduce the swelling. Occasionally, your doctor may prescribe a diuretic (also called a water pill) to help your body get rid of extra fluid by making you urinate.

You can also retain fluid if you have small tumors in the abdomen from metastatic cancer. This fluid buildup can cause swelling and discomfort. We call this ascites. This condition can decrease over time with treatment, but some patients may benefit from having fluid removed through a procedure called a paracentesis. To do this, a doctor will insert a thin needle or catheter into the abdomen to drain excess fluid. Sometimes a doctor will use ultrasound to find the best place to insert the needle or catheter.

Causes of Weight Loss

There are two main reasons for patients to show dramatic weight loss during the course of breast cancer treatment. The first of these covers a broad group of digestive issues caused by the cancer or the chemotherapy that make eating less appealing or that make digestion less efficient. You may feel less like eating because of nausea, because the taste of food has changed, or because your digestive process has slowed. In rare cases, you may have a mass blocking the digestive tract in some way that makes eating uncomfortable. Most of these situations are treatable. The other major reason for weight loss in patients with metastatic cancer is something called anorexia-cachexia, and researchers don't know exactly what causes it. It is a progressive weight loss triggered by the cancer itself, and it is not yet treatable beyond just treating the cancer.

I discuss anorexia-cachexia in a little more detail later in this chapter, but it tends to be less common among patients with advanced breast cancer, as compared to patients with other types of advanced cancer. When you come to your doctor asking about how to put weight on or keep it on, you have to know that your medical team can treat some of the issues that contribute to weight loss but not all of them. I can give you some strategies to use, along with help from your doctor, to stimulate your appetite and take in more calories (table 13.1), but some weight loss is hard to treat. Some of its causes have been addressed in other chapters, and we address several more in this chapter. A few that may be unfamiliar to you are mucositis (inflammation or sores in the mouth and throat), difficulty swallowing, and lactose insufficiency. These are easily treatable in most cases, and, in the case of mucositis, we can treat the pain until the symptoms go away, at which point eating will be more enjoyable again.

Table 13.1. Treatment options for underlying causes of weight loss

Factors that contribute to decreased appetite and weight loss	Possible treatment options
Nausea	Determine the cause of the nausea and aggressively treat (see chapter 9).
Decreased appetite	Dietary changes, appetite stimulants
Constipation	Goal for bowel movement every day or every other day. Use stimulant laxatives to ensure bowels are moving appropriately (see chapter 10).
Changes in taste and smell	Dietary changes, wait it out
Early satiety (getting full quickly)	Dietary changes, treat gastroparesis
Gastroparesis (slow movement of food in stomach)	Use medications that encourage movement of food through the GI tract (e.g., metoclopramide) (see chapter 10).
Depression	Treat depression with antidepressants that are known to stimulate weight gain (e.g., mirtazapine) (see chapter 17).
Mucositis	Treat pain associated with the mucositis.

Mucositis and Throat Pain

You might already know that chemotherapy can cause mucositis, sores, or thrush in the mouth or throat. If you have pain when you swallow, this is called odynophagia, and its potential causes include infection, chemotherapy agents, or radiation. Thrush, or oral candidiasis, is a fungal (yeast) infection of the mouth that can be triggered by the steroids you are taking for nausea or the side effects of cancer. It creates white, cottage cheese–like spots on the tongue and mouth. Or if it occurs deeper in the throat, you will notice pain when swallowing. This can be treated with antifungal mouthwashes, such as nystatin. If this doesn't work, or if it tastes too awful, you can take an oral antifungal called fluconazole that comes in either pill or liquid form. Typically, this kind of infection clears up within 48 hours.

Mucositis is harder to treat, but we can reduce the pain while the sores are healing. Your doctor may suggest an oral rinse that will numb the pain and make it easier to eat meals. Oncologists often refer to these rinses as "magic mouthwash," and the recipes for magic mouthwash can vary. Most contain viscous lidocaine, which numbs the nerves of the mouth. It's similar to what your dentist might use before a procedure. Many oral rinses contain lidocaine, Kaopectate, or Benadryl that you swish around in your mouth and then swallow to take away any pain in your mouth and throat. This won't cure the sores—only time will do that—but it will keep the pain at bay. If the pain is severe, you may need additional pain medication. And if you've had cold sores in the past or oral herpes, you may need antiviral medications to treat these sores, which may also emerge after chemotherapy.

Another common tactic is to avoid foods that will exacerbate the sores. That means no hot and spicy foods, alcohol, or sodas. Also avoid acidic foods, including citrus juices, and coarse foods, including chips, crusty breads, and raw vegetables.

Finally, you want to keep drinking lots of fluids all day long. If you are eating less, you still need to stay hydrated. And you should feel reassured that mucositis and mouth sores will resolve over the course of several days. They come and go with the cycles of chemotherapy. If they are becoming a problem that is affecting the quality of your life, then lowering the dose of chemotherapy is one way to reduce the severity of mucositis.

Lactose Intolerance

As we age, our stomachs lose the ability to make the enzyme lactase, which breaks down the sugars in dairy products. Some chemotherapies also interfere with lactase production or exacerbate the normal, progressive lactose intolerance that we all develop over time. All this means is you may start to have difficulty digesting dairy products (if you weren't already lactose intolerant). You don't want to be dealing with bloating and diarrhea if you are trying to put on weight or keep it on. So if this happens, you can take lactase pills to alleviate the problem whenever you're eating a dairy product.

Strategies for Keeping Weight On

Many people spend part of their adult lives trying to lose weight by restricting calories, eating salads and other foods that have low caloric density, and avoiding snacks and high-fat foods. When you try to gain or maintain a weight, you have to reverse most of that logic. It sounds fairly simple. The wrinkle is that there will be some days when you want to eat but don't feel up to it, and there might be some foods that you used to love that don't taste right anymore. In fact, even the smell of certain foods might give you an unpleasant reaction. So you have to experiment a little to see what foods you like and what you can safely eat.

Try a wide variety of foods. Some people who used to love sweets find that they really want only savory foods while in treatment. Some people who used to hate spicy foods find them suddenly more appealing. Try new foods to see what works.

Take care of your teeth. Oral hygiene really matters when you are dealing with dysgeusia, which is the change in the way foods taste after chemotherapy. Not every patient experiences this. If you do, you need to brush your teeth and tongue every day and floss to keep the problem from getting worse. For whatever reason, dysgeusia tends to improve over time. Doctors call this effect the tincture of time. Either you adjust to the new taste of food, or the effect itself wears off after some time.

Pay attention to calories. If you have advanced, progressive breast cancer and are struggling to gain weight, your goal is to take in as many calories as you can each day. The good news is that there are a lot of calories in butter and soy and full-fat dairy products, as well as nuts and nut butters, so if you can tolerate those, you can include more high-fat foods in your diet than other people usually can.

Eat more frequently. Larger meals three times a day are probably not an option when your appetite is not what it normally is. I tell people to eat small meals throughout the day. Your goal is to snack all day in hopes of accumulating enough calories over time. Don't be discouraged if you can eat just a few bites at a time. In fact, people feel better when they start with an extremely small portion and then take more if they are still hungry. Sometimes facing a huge plate of food is discouraging.

Try energy drink supplements. You can buy these at the store or make your own smoothies with whatever you want—full-fat ice cream, chocolate protein powder. It's up to you. If you can't tolerate milk-based products or don't like the taste of them, you can try some juice-based products or make your own juice smoothies.

Be careful about fiber. Some people who are struggling with constipation may need fiber in their diet to keep things moving, while others who are struggling with loose stools may find that salads and bran products exacerbate the problem. Some patients who loved salads can no longer enjoy them while in treatment. Others are thrilled to say no, finally, to bran muffins.

Avoiding Guilt Trips

Vicki encourages people to practice self-compassion while they are finding new ways to eat. That also means urging family members to be careful about pushing food on cancer patients for their own good. People actually struggle more with eating when they feel pressured. The last thing you want is to have the dinner table become a battleground—even if it's done out of love. One patient, Martha, said that her daughter would whip up batches of her famous pudding and then feed it to her by the spoonful, as though she was a toddler. She finally put up her hand and said, "Stop. If I am hungry, I'll eat more." Of course, her daughter was hurt and afraid that if she didn't make her mother eat, she wasn't being a good caretaker.

Patients who are losing weight in treatment know that they should eat more, but they are struggling with all kinds of difficulties, including nausea, pain, and lack of appetite or even an aversion to food. Sometimes they need to eat very small meals, such as a quarter of a muffin or a few bites of pasta, or they are afraid they will make themselves sick. From the outside, that doesn't seem like enough food. But it's better to respect the patient and to encourage eating without making them feel bad if they can't. It's not realistic to expect cancer patients to eat the way they did before. Sometimes your loved one will want to sit at the table and enjoy the conversation without eating much, and that has to be okay. I tell family members to offer foods they like to eat and leave the rest up to them.

In the palliative care clinic, I met Moira, a colleague's patient with metastatic breast cancer who had progressed through several treatments. Her daughter began the visit by expressing her distress over feeling that her mother wasn't eating enough. Moira was at a normal weight and appeared healthy but told me that she was used to be being much heavier and felt really uncomfortable with how much weight she had lost. None of her clothes fit anymore. She said she didn't look or feel like herself and was trying to eat normally, but she didn't feel hungry. She was tearful because she wasn't tempted by any of her favorite foods. It was one more sign that she wasn't herself, and she feared that her appetite would never return. What made things worse was the constant nagging from family members that she should be eating more.

As a patient, you want to be clear with your family that you aren't rejecting the food itself or the love of the people who made it. Educate yourself about nutrition and experiment with eating different foods you might like in small portions several times a day. Also try to be with those you love when they are eating even if you aren't feeling like eating too much yourself. Meals are such a significant social time for most families. When weight loss is persistent, everyone needs to remember that you aren't eating less because you're giving up, but rather it is the body's response to the cancer. Preserve meals as a social time to enjoy each other's company.

Appetite Stimulants

Some people are really bothered by their lack of appetite and want to know whether any medications will help. Appetite stimulants don't help patients with metastatic disease (cancer that has spread) to live longer, but some people just want to eat more because they want to feel more normal. That's a good enough reason to give them a try, but be aware of the burdens and benefits of each medication first.

Dronabinol is a synthetic cannabinoid that can increase appetite, but it often needs to be taken several times a day. Some patients experience a high with this medication, which some find pleasant and others find disorienting. I don't like recommending cannabinoids to people who have a history of psychiatric illness or dementia or who are elderly because I worry about the risk of confusion and anxiety. We caution patients that marijuana and its chemical constituents aren't a cure-all and you should discuss any use with your clinicians.

Olanzapine is an antipsychotic medication that was created as a treatment for patients with confusion or thought disorders, but there is evidence that it is a powerful antinausea medication (chapter 9) and may also stimulate appetite and weight gain.

Mirtazapine is an antidepressant and sleep medication that also stimulates hunger in low doses.

Megestrol acetate contains progesterone and can be helpful to stimulate appetite in some people. However, it can also contribute to blood clots. Many physicians will avoid this medication.

Steroids as Appetite Stimulants

Steroids are chemicals that your body already makes in the adrenal glands. Giving additional doses of prednisone or dexamethasone can stimulate both appetite and energy. Even a very low dose of dexamethasone (1 milligram per day) can relieve fatigue and stimulate hunger. I had a patient, Delores, who was on a regimen of chemo that required dexamethasone to be given for a day before each infusion and a day after. This is a common antinausea and antiallergy treatment with some chemotherapy. She said to me that she loved those preinfusion days when she was on steroids. She ate nearly full-sized meals and felt like "the Energizer bunny." Then she switched to a new line of chemo that didn't require steroids. One day in the clinic, she whispered, "What do I have to do to get my hands on some more of that dexamethasone? Thanksgiving is coming and I want to eat!"

Whenever patients ask questions like this, I always want to know more about how they truly feel while taking the drug in question. I ask because there are a lot of unpleasant immediate side effects with steroids, including irritability, anxiety or depression, difficulty sleeping, fluid retention, and difficulty controlling blood sugar. Long-term side effects include weight gain, fat deposits in the abdomen and face, muscle weakness, high blood pressure, stomach irritation, and osteoporosis. Even though these side effects tend to occur at higher doses, you can see why doctors are reluctant to prescribe steroids as a long-term solution for patients who just want to eat a bit more.

Still, some patients don't experience any of the difficult side effects at very low doses when they use the medication cautiously. I prescribed Delores 1 milligram of dexamethasone as needed and told her how sparingly I thought it should be used. She took it the day of Thanksgiving, Christmas Eve, and Christmas Day. At her next appointment, she told me how much she ate and how wonderful it was to feel like herself at the dinner table on those special days.

Anorexia-Cachexia

You might continue to lose weight even if you do everything you can to eat enough calories and stimulate your appetite. One major cause of weight loss in patients with metastatic cancer is anorexia-cachexia syndrome, which I mentioned earlier. Anorexia means "lack of appetite for food," and cachexia refers to significant loss of weight and muscle mass.

People with certain cancers, such as lung and pancreatic cancers, have a higher incidence of this syndrome. It occurs less commonly in patients with breast cancer. Researchers don't yet fully understand what triggers this weight loss, but the suspicion is that some tumors contribute to a production of proteins called cytokines. These cytokines have complicated names, such as interleukin-6 and tumor necrosis factor alpha, and they appear to speed up the body's metabolism while also decreasing appetite. They can also prevent the body from absorbing nutrients from the foods you do eat. All of these factors make anorexia-cachexia progressive in nature.

Unfortunately, it's also hard to treat. Offering nutrition through a feeding tube inserted into the stomach or intestines or through an IV does not help with weight loss from anorexia cachexia in advanced cancer. It also won't help to improve survival or quality of life. For these reasons, many doctors will not recommend a feeding tube or an IV for artificial nutrition.

Sometimes patients and families come to the clinic to ask about progressive weight loss when really they are asking a much bigger question about how treatment is going. Weight loss is one of the universal signs that the cancer might be advancing, and it can trigger a lot of worry. When a patient or family member becomes adamant about artificial nutrition or putting on weight, I know that they are often worrying about what this means for them. Patients sometimes start to ask questions about the cancer progressing. This is a good time to start talking with your clinicians about several issues. I like asking patients things like, "What is your body telling you?," "What are your concerns about the future?," and "What is good quality of life for you right now?" Many times, people are relieved to give voice to these concerns and to talk about what they truly want for themselves.

Medical Marijuana

I mentioned the synthetic cannabinoid dronabinol earlier, and doctors are often also asked about the use of medical marijuana in the setting of cancer treatment. Clinicians have varying opinions on this subject. Some consider the studies of marijuana to treat pain and nausea very compelling, while others worry that the studies that have been done do not show that it is efficacious or even safe for all patients. Unfortunately, there is no proof behind any of the healing claims with regard to cancer.

Marijuana is a product of the cannabis plant, and the active ingredient is tetrahydrocannabinol, or THC. But THC is one of only hundreds of compounds in marijuana, including many different cannabinoids (the active chemicals in marijuana), and there is conflicting medical data about what any of them can or can't do. Marijuana has some antinausea, antianxiety, appetite-stimulant, and pain-reducing qualities, but there is little clinical data to help guide doctors in helping patients make decisions on how to apply its use.

The other challenge with marijuana is that it's not the best drug for relieving any of the major symptoms in the cancer setting, including nausea, pain, anorexia, or anxiety. Actually, its effect on any of these symptoms can vary greatly from individual to individual. Some people swear by marijuana, and almost every cancer patient has been approached by a well-intentioned friend or family member who pleads with them to try it. Many times, people who used and enjoyed marijuana before they got cancer continue to use it to good effect after their diagnosis. Even those people who have never used it before may find some value in it once they have a diagnosis. Most doctors are not opposed to the idea of trying it, and you may find it helpful.

Nutritional Supplements

Lots of patients tell me that they have begun to use various health foods, alternative therapies, and nutritional supplements to augment the cancer treatments they are getting. There is an enormous number of nutritional supplements marketed as cures or preventive measures for every kind of ailment, including cancer. Cumulatively, patients have given me a long list of products they are taking and alternate therapies they have tried, including coenzyme Q; turmeric; milk thistle; mushroom extracts; coffee enemas; shark cartilage; high doses of vitamins C, E, and A; and teas of every kind. In some cases they just tell me what they are taking, and in other cases they ask me what I think of these supplements. Will they help?

I know my fellow oncologists get these questions, too, and they worry about how to respond. Some oncologists tell me that they just shrug and change the subject. Dave, Vicki and I like to keep the lines of communication open on this subject, because your medical team needs to know what you are taking and at what doses.

I tell patients that some herbs and supplements do have a pharmacological effect on the body, meaning they can dilute or change the effect of the medications you may be taking to control nausea or pain or other symptoms of cancer—or even the cancer therapy itself. At higher doses, some of them also bring their own side effects, such as a sensitivity in the skin to light, which is a problem for people undergoing radiation, or digestive trouble, or they may even function as anticoagulants in the blood. This is what I tell patients:

- Keep your oncologist and your medical team apprised of what you are taking and at what doses. I suggest that patients bring in a list of any supplements that they may be taking, or even photos of the labels on the bottles. I often run this list by our pharmacist to see if there are concerns about how the supplements may interact with a person's breast cancer therapies. Sometimes supplements have estrogenic properties, which we recommend avoiding in patients with a history of breast cancer as well.

- Stay aware of any changes in your body and how you are feeling. You want to report any new side effects or possible interactions between these supplemental therapies and your current medication.

- Keep a critical eye on the science behind the claims for cancer cures. Some websites cite studies that were poorly designed or that have since been disputed.

Also, it's important to talk to your doctor about whether you are thinking about taking supplements or alternative therapies in addition to or instead of the cancer therapies that your team may recommend. I care for a woman in her forties with metastatic breast cancer who declined standard cancer therapy and was instead taking various supplements. When I asked her about her hopes and expectations with respect to the supplements, she said she felt more in control and that she was advised by her naturopath that these supplements would cure her of the cancer. I was honest with her about my worry that the cancer would progress more rapidly without standard therapies and my concern that the supplements would not provide the cure she hoped for. I also tell my patients that as their oncologist, I will always care for them—whether they decide to take the therapies I recommend or not. One of the worst things about having cancer is that sense that you can't control the outcome. Sometimes simply voicing these concerns can provide enormous relief for ongoing anxiety. By contrast, taking large numbers of supplements can give the illusion of control without allowing you to talk about and address your actual concerns.

CHAPTER FOURTEEN

What If I Have a Sudden Fever?

Everyone in a cancer clinic seems obsessed with the idea of preventing infection. There are posters everywhere telling you to notify the receptionist if you have a fever or a cough. And you probably notice the way everyone is using the hand sanitizers mounted outside each exam room and along the hallways. There are good reasons for all of this concern, and your doctors will talk to you about your risk of infection and what symptoms to look for.

Chemotherapy and other cancer treatments can affect your immune system by lowering the rate of neutrophils in your blood, which are the body's first line of defense against infection. These cells help your body kill or neutralize the normally occurring bacteria on your skin, in your mouth and lungs, and in your digestive tract and keep them from entering your bloodstream. As your rate of neutrophils goes down, you are at increased risk of developing infection from bacteria that already exist in your system. Also, cancer cells can sometimes invade tissues and organs in a way that makes infection more likely to develop. In some cases, the port inserted to make chemotherapy infusions easier can become a site of infection. Although a developing infection is a serious condition that requires medical attention, it's something that your cancer team is used to dealing with and is usually easily treatable.

In this chapter, I (Dave) describe the signs of infection, how your doctor will try to discover the source of the infection, and how most infections are treated. Patients who are receiving a certain type of targeted therapy called immunotherapy are also at higher risk of developing certain types of infections, and you should know about those.

Risk of Infection

Ask your doctor about your risk of infection; not every breast cancer patient will be at high risk as the result of treatment. The patients who are at higher risk are those who

- have had a recent surgery;
- are on chemotherapy; or
- are being treated for metastatic breast cancer with treatments that may lower your white blood cell count.

Many patients with breast cancer are at no higher risk than an average person for developing an infection. For example, early-stage breast cancer patients who are on hormonal therapy are at no increased risk of infection from treatment. So, if you are in this category, you won't need to call your oncologist or medical team to report every fever.

Signs of Fever and Other Symptoms of Infection

If you are at a higher risk of developing infection from treatment, you should always call your doctor if you have a temperature of 100.5 degrees Fahrenheit or higher or have shaking chills. This is true even if you feel relatively fine. The higher your fever, the more serious your infection can be. Your doctor will need to know about your symptoms to determine whether you might need to come in to the clinic. In some cases, we send patients directly to the emergency room. While you might just have the common cold, your team needs to make sure it's not something more serious.

If you have chills that cause you to shake, you may be starting to spike a fever. If you have shaking chills, take your temperature right away and then take it again after 15 minutes.

Other signs of infection include the following:

- Unexpected redness and tenderness on your skin
- Painful urination, which could be a urinary tract infection
- Cough or difficulty breathing
- Sudden onset of confusion, particularly in elderly patients for whom confusion may be the only overt sign of infection

These are the most common signs of infection, but if you have any new symptoms, you will want to share them with your doctor. The daughter of one of my patients called me to say that her mother was acting strangely. She was taking a longer time to answer questions and seemed mildly confused. We asked her to come in for an evaluation, and I admitted her to the hospital out of concern that she could have had a stroke. Then she spiked a temperature, and her chest x-ray showed signs of a pneumonia. After she started on antibiotics, her fevers went away, and her confusion disappeared.

Some people may be at higher risk for developing infection during treatment if they've had recurring infections in the past. Vicki had a patient who was just starting to be treated for breast cancer. She felt great during treatment and told Vicki that, aside from the infusions, she could hardly believe she had cancer. On about the ninth day after her third infusion, she told her husband she was suddenly tired and wanted a nap. An hour later, her husband found her asleep and drenched in sweat. He checked her temperature, and it was 102 degrees. She called the clinic and came in immediately to have her blood drawn. The attending doctor ordered antibiotics for her even before the blood work came back, and when it did come back, it indicated that she had the start of what would have been a runaway infection. Later the patient told Vicki that she'd had a history of urinary tract infections, particularly after sex. So Vicki's sensible advice was to mark a calendar for the seventh, eighth, and ninth days after each infusion and to refrain from sex on those days because the risk of infection is greatest on these days.

Getting Treatment

Infections can be caused by three types of organisms: bacteria, viruses, and fungi. If you have a bacterial infection, which is the most common type, you'll take antibiotics to kill the offending bacteria. Viruses, such as herpes or shingles, are treated with antivirals, and you may be more prone to reinfection from recurring viruses while in cancer treatment. Fungal infections are not common in patients with breast cancer. However, they can occur if patients are being treated with chemotherapy or are on a prolonged course of steroids. Thrush, a fungal infection, can show up as white plaques in the mouth or further down in the esophagus. These can be treated with antifungal dissolving tablets or solutions.

It can be tempting to dismiss a slight fever or nagging cough or the sudden onset of fatigue and chills because these seem insignificant compared to many of the other side effects of cancer treatment. It's tempting for anyone to want to take acetaminophen (Tylenol), put on a sweater, or have a nap in hopes of feeling better in a couple of hours. But cancer is notorious for triggering infections inside the body, and even a small infection can get out of control in a hurry. You can get dangerously sick within a couple of days. If uncontrolled, you can develop sepsis, a condition in which bacteria is in your blood stream and causes your blood pressure to drop quickly. At that point, you can die of infection. By contrast, if you call the clinic, sit through a blood test, and find out that you really do just have a virus, no one will be upset.

Can I Catch Infection?

People with cancer are always worried about whether they can catch infections from friends, family, or being out in a crowd, and sometimes they ask whether they need to wear a mask. For most patients with cancer, your ability to catch these routine viral infections is about the same as it is for those who don't have cancer. Of course, getting a cold or a flu is not fun even when you are perfectly healthy, and new respiratory illnesses may emerge. With COVID-19, oncologists were initiating tailored discussions with patients about their relative risks for getting sick and what precautions they might take to minimize their risk. Talk to your doctor about what your risks are, and whether you need to take additional precautions to stay healthy. It's important to get your flu shots and other vaccines, and to follow public health guidelines about wearing masks. Use your good judgment in avoiding people who are sick and keep hand sanitizer with you while you are out and interacting with other people.

You may wonder, too, whether you need to take antibiotics before any dental procedures or teeth cleaning. Usually that's not necessary unless you have a known heart murmur and have always taken this precaution. Theoretically though, any hardware inside your body, such as a portacath, can become infected after a dental procedure or cleaning. Take the same precautions of noticing and reporting any new symptoms that may arise.

Blood Tests and Infection

The main reason your medical team will be closely monitoring your blood counts during every chemotherapy treatment is to monitor your risk of infection. Your level of white blood cells will decrease in the days following each infusion, and you should know that you are more prone to infection about seven to ten days after an infusion, when your white blood count will be lowest. Some other treatments may also decrease your white blood cells, including the CDK4/6 inhibitors. These treatments will also require regular blood tests.

You can ask your doctor about the level of neutrophils in your complete blood count. This is called the absolute neutrophil count, or ANC. This level reveals your underlying risk of infection. Even if your level of neutrophils is high enough for you to continue with your treatment, you can still be vulnerable to infection afterward since the ANC usually drops with treatment.

Neutropenia

When your white blood count is low, you may not have many signs of an infection. Sometimes the only sign is fever. This is known as febrile neutropenia. All the other signs of infection—cough, redness, swelling, or pain—are caused by the white blood cells infiltrating an area in an attempt to fight the infection. When cancer therapies lower your white blood count, there aren't enough cells to create these other symptoms. That's why getting medical attention immediately is critical. Without treatment, bacteria from the infected area can get into the bloodstream, causing blood infections such as sepsis, septicemia, or bacteremia, which are all medical emergencies.

Thankfully, most cases of febrile neutropenia are easily treated. Most episodes respond well to antibiotics. And if you are at high risk for developing infection, your doctor may prescribe growth factors, which are medications that help boost your neutrophil count.

If you are being treated with chemotherapy, there will be predictable times during the chemotherapy cycle when you are most at risk for neutropenia. As noted earlier, for most regimens this occurs seven to ten days after the chemotherapy was administered. Chemotherapy regimens that are given weekly may hold a lower risk of infection because the white blood count doesn't get that low.

Hormonal agents, such as tamoxifen and the aromatase inhibitors, don't carry a significant risk of bone marrow suppression and thus don't carry a significant risk of lowering white blood cell count. Therefore, women with early-stage breast cancer being treated with hormonal therapies like tamoxifen and the aromatase inhibitors are not considered at an increased risk for serious infection. However, those patients with metastatic breast cancer who are being treated with hormonal therapy and a CDK4/6 inhibitor are at risk for neutropenia. That's why they will have frequent blood tests, particularly in the first weeks after treatment starts.

You can ask your oncologist whether the risk of infection for your specific treatment is low, medium, or high. For patients at high risk of infection, we will often use growth factors to spur on the bone marrow to make more white blood cells.

More About Cancer Treatments That Cause Infection

It's possible for you to develop an infection as the result of a recent surgery. Sometimes, an infection can develop under the tissue as it heals. In that case, you might have to go back into the hospital and have a surgeon reopen the incision to allow the pus to drain directly out of the wound. If you have a breast implant in place, it may need to be removed and replaced, sometimes at a later date.

Another possible source of infection when patients are on chemotherapy is the catheters and medical hardware that we put in patients to help treat the cancer. For example, the skin overlying the portacath can become infected. Stents that we put into the GI tract or the ureters can become infected from the bacteria in your bowel, or ureters when the white count gets too low. That's why your doctor will ask you whether you have any catheters, stents, or hardware when you have an infection.

Immunotherapy treatments use the body's own immune system to help kill cancer cells. For decades, researchers studied cancer cells in isolation, wondering why they grow and mutate the way they do. Recently, researchers have focused on the fact that cancer cells don't exist in isolation. They interact with the body's other systems, including the immune system. New research focuses on the ways in which certain cancer cells can essentially fool the immune system into leaving them alone instead of killing them off as defective. This research has yielded some dramatic success stories in particular types of cancer and has shown results in some types of breast cancer. As noted in chapter 4, immunotherapy is now being used along with chemotherapy to treat metastatic triple-negative breast cancer.

One downside is that newly empowered immune cells may attack healthy tissues as well. For example, in the tissues in the colon this can cause infections that mimic colitis. If you are undergoing immuno-therapy, your doctor will talk to you about the risks of developing these secondary infections and how to manage them.

CHAPTER FIFTEEN

Clotting and Bleeding Issues

The process of clotting and bleeding in your body is an intense balancing act that goes on throughout your life. You don't usually notice it unless you have a cut or a scrape. You have proteins continually circulating in your system with the sole purpose of patrolling for breaks in the vascular system. When you do get a cut on your hand, for example, platelets arrive at the site of the cut first to plug it, and then clotting factors—proteins responsible for knitting the clot—layer on top of these platelets. Within minutes, the clot has stopped the bleeding.

If a clot continued to grow, it would clog the blood vessel entirely, and then the tissues on the other side of it wouldn't get the oxygen and nutrients they need. So the body has a competing system of proteins that dissolve clots and prevent them from becoming too big. In medical terms, this process of dissolving clots is called lysis.

As you can imagine, both cancer and cancer treatment can upset this careful balance in the body between clotting and lysis, which is why your doctors will be concerned about the risks of bleeding or developing clots while you are in treatment. Your medical team will have a lot of experience in managing these issues.

The Risk of Blood Clots

Cancers can secrete proteins that make it easier for the blood to form clots. This means that patients with cancer, particularly metastatic cancers, are more likely to develop blood clots than someone without cancer. I (Jenn) have been caring for Alanna, a 71-year-old woman with HER2-positive metastatic breast cancer. A few months ago, she came in for routine CT scans. Alanna has been doing great in treatment, and we expected the scans to reflect this. After she left, I was paged by the radiology team because Alanna's scans showed a pulmonary embolus, or blood clot, in her lungs. A blood clot in the lungs is a medical emergency (see table 2.1 on page 26), so I immediately called Alanna to check in with her. She was surprised to hear about the clot because she was feeling fine and not experiencing any relevant symptoms. She had no shortness of breath or chest pain. I asked her to come back to the clinic immediately, and we started her on blood thinners that day because whenever we find a clot, we always worry that another, larger blood clot might develop. You may need to be admitted to the hospital for further evaluation and treatment for a blood clot if you have symptoms or low oxygen or blood pressure.

If you develop a blood clot, your doctor will probably start you on a blood thinner, like we did with Alanna. Typically, this involves giving yourself a shot under the skin once or twice a day, just as you would if you were a diabetic who needed to self-inject insulin. There are also oral drugs, such as apixaban, that may be an option for you.

Less frequently, there may be a blood clot in the lungs that impacts the pumping function of the heart, causing low blood pressure. If this is the case, sometimes the clot can be removed. Or your doctor may use something called a tissue plasminogen activator to dissolve a clot.

What Symptoms Can I Look For?

While many patients like Alanna do not have any symptoms of a blood clot in their lungs, there are some things to look out for. People who have a pulmonary embolus may experience shortness of breath, chest discomfort, particularly when taking in a deep breath, or cough. People may also experience lightheadedness and dizziness or feel like they are fainting, but this is rare. If you experience any of these symptoms, call your clinic right away. Your doctor may want to order a chest scan to see if there is a problem.

Sometimes blood clots form in the legs and then move to the lungs. A blood clot in the leg is called a deep vein thrombosis, or DVT. The most common symptoms of DVT is a noticeable swelling or tenderness in one leg or discomfort in the calf, though not everyone experiences this. If you do, you want to call the clinic immediately because there is a risk that part of the clot can break away and settle in the lungs. Your doctor may recommend coming to the clinic for an ultrasound to see if the swelling is a DVT.

Tamoxifen and Blood Clots

If you have early-stage hormone receptor–positive breast cancer, you may be treated with tamoxifen. This medication is sometimes prescribed for advanced cancer as well. Tamoxifen can slightly increase your risk of developing a blood clot, and while it's not common (a five-year risk of around 1%) it's important to be aware of this possible risk. If you are undergoing an elective surgery, talk to your doctor about whether you need to hold off on the tamoxifen in the days before and after surgery. Surgery that requires bed rest or that will reduce your activity level can also increase your risk of developing blood clots, and tamoxifen may add to this risk a little bit.

We've all heard that people can be at increased risk of developing DVT while on long flights or drives. Women taking tamoxifen often ask about their risk in these scenarios as well. I tell them that it's a good idea for anyone to take regular breaks to walk around and stretch while traveling.

The Risk of Bleeding

Sometimes chemotherapy can prevent your bone marrow from making enough platelets, or perhaps the cancer itself is destroying the platelets. Remember that platelets are like the marines. They're the first ones to attack. They will stop any major bleeding by laying down the initial aspects of a clot. If you don't have enough platelets or they are not functioning properly, your body will have a hard time forming a blood clot. If this happens, you may have frequent nosebleeds or even see blood in your stool.

Most times when platelet counts are low, the bleeding caused isn't terribly serious, but if your level of platelets gets below 10,000 per microliter, doctors start to worry about the risk of bleeding into the brain. Thankfully, dropping this low is very rare. If it happens, we can give platelet transfusions to raise the level, and that usually stops the bleeding. Platelet transfusions are effective for a day or two, and in the meantime your doctor will be working to figure out the underlying cause. For example, if the cancer itself is causing the body to create an antibody that destroys the platelets, the best form of treatment is chemotherapy to kill the cancer. As the tumor cells die, your platelet count will rebound.

Blood Transfusions

You may benefit from a blood transfusion if your body is struggling to produce enough red blood cells or platelets because your bone marrow function has been suppressed from cancer treatments. Patients who do need one often ask whether they are at risk for developing infections from donated blood, but the reality is that this procedure is very safe. In a transfusion, you are receiving blood from volunteer donors, but blood banks carefully screen blood. So the risk of getting HIV from a blood transfusion is 1 in 2.1 million. The risk of being exposed to hepatitis B is about 1 in 275,000, and the risk of hepatitis C is 1 in 1.9 million. All of these risks are extremely low.

What your medical team will be concerned about is the risk of allergic reaction, which sometimes comes in the form of a fever or rash. Before we administer blood, we always check your ABO blood type and administer the same type of blood. But there are other proteins of lesser importance that are present on the surface of red blood cells, and an allergic reaction can happen when your body is incompatible with one or more of these lesser proteins and your immune system attacks the red blood cells. In rare instances, this reaction can cause lung injury or other complications. That's why your doctors and nurses will be monitoring your reaction to the transfusion as it happens and for several days afterward, looking for any signs of an adverse reaction. At the first sign of a problem, they will stop the transfusion and treat you for the reaction. Even if this happens, most patients fully recover.

Some people ask whether they can have a friend or family member donate blood to limit the risks of an adverse reaction or infection. You can do this, but there is no evidence that these donations are safer than pooled volunteer donations. In fact, some hospitals discourage these direct donations, however heartfelt, because of the time and effort required to test the blood after it has been collected. All donations, regardless of source, must be screened for infections, including HIV and hepatitis, before they can be used. And donors have to go through the same screening process and questionnaire that they would at a blood bank, and they may have to submit to this process more than once. While friends and family may say that they are eager to help, most doctors have found that this process introduces delays and stress into a situation that is already emotionally fraught. If friends and family members do want to donate blood as a sign of support, they can do so at a blood bank, knowing that they may be saving someone else's life.

CHAPTER SIXTEEN

Why Am I So Exhausted?
When Will I Have Energy Again?

Fatigue is one of the most common symptoms patients experience while in cancer treatment and something we address with all patients in the palliative care clinic. Cancer fatigue is not like any kind of exhaustion that you've experienced before. It might not improve much with rest or a good night's sleep. In fact, some patients refer to fatigue as an unwanted partner in treatment and complain that it, more than anything, makes them feel isolated from family and from the life they used to lead. Some fatigue after each treatment is expected; you may not feel able to do more than rest and sleep in the days following an infusion. This is normal and your energy level should rebound day by day.

Someone on your medical team should ask you about your general level of fatigue at every visit to the clinic. The National Comprehensive Cancer Network publishes guidelines for oncologists on how to provide the best treatment and for patients on how to get the best care, and they encourage patients to keep an open dialog with doctors about fatigue at every infusion because it can so deeply affect quality of life. You might want to keep notes, similar to the notes that you keep on other side effects, so that you can describe your energy level after each treatment and how quickly it rebounds.

Doctors often use a visual analog scale similar to the one for tracking pain, so you will be asked to rate your fatigue on a scale of 0 to 10. Zero means no fatigue at all and 10 indicates the worst fatigue you can ever imagine. Keeping track of how you feel day by day will help your doctors determine whether you are having the episodic fatigue common after an infusion or whether your fatigue is ongoing, which may be caused by other factors, such as medication, sleeplessness, depression, or the cancer itself.

The key is to ask your doctor about any reversible causes and develop strategies to manage your energy effectively. This might involve taking different pain medications, working to get a better night's sleep, or addressing any anxiety or underlying depression. In this chapter, I (Vicki) will go over the most common causes of cancer-related fatigue and strategies to lessen the effects on your day-to-day life.

Episodic Fatigue

If you have early-stage breast cancer, there are several treatments that can cause severe, but temporary, fatigue. For example, you might expect to feel exhausted in the days and weeks after surgery. Radiation treatments also cause fatigue. This surprises some people because the treatment is focused on such a small area of the body. Fatigue from radiation can be cumulative, meaning that in a series of radiation treatments, you can expect to feel more exhausted in the final treatments than you did after the first round of radiation. And most people know that chemotherapy causes fatigue that can last for several days, or even a week.

Women with metastatic breast cancer also experience episodic fatigue in treatment. They may feel exhausted in the days after an infusion and then recover their energy in the days leading to their next infusion. Or, they may be on cycles of oral agents like palbociclib and may feel better whenever they have a week off of treatment.

In all of these cases, the fatigue may feel extreme but remember that it's temporary. As the days pass, your energy level will increase and you will feel more like yourself again.

Hormonal Treatments and Fatigue

Many patients report to me that they are experiencing fatigue while taking hormonal treatments for breast cancer. It's always challenging to figure out if the hormonal therapy is directly causing fatigue or if some other factor may be the cause. If a woman has just completed surgery or radiation therapy and started on hormonal therapy, the fatigue may be more related to the recovery from the surgery or radiation. There are so many factors that can contribute to fatigue, including anxiety, insomnia, and lack of exercise. For example, if you are experiencing hot flashes at night, you may not be getting enough quality sleep. Your oncologist may involve your primary care doctor as well to make sure that there are no other medical reasons for feeling persistently tired, such as low thyroid function.

If you are taking hormonal treatments for breast cancer, you should report fatigue to your oncologist or someone on your medical team because we want to know how you are doing in general, and we may be able to help. Jenn just saw a woman in follow-up who thought that her anastrozole was causing significant fatigue, but when treated with a medication at bedtime to help with her nocturnal hot flashes, she slept better and was delighted to find that her energy level rebounded.

Ongoing Fatigue

There are going to be some days during treatment where you expect to be tired. If you know that the first two days after an infusion are the ones when you feel wiped out, the fatigue is more manageable because you can sort of wait it out. I'm more concerned about ongoing fatigue, in which your energy level seems to lag for weeks. If you have fatigue like this that doesn't improve for several days or affects your quality of life in a consistent way, then your care team needs to know. If you were my patient, the first question I would ask is what you want to be doing that you can't do because of the fatigue. Those answers are really revealing. The person who says, "I can't do anything because I feel that I need to sleep all day," is dealing with a totally different problem than the patient who says, "I used to get through thirty-six holes of golf, and now I can barely do eighteen." If you can't do everything that you used to do, you may be setting expectations too high for yourself while in treatment. By contrast, if you can't do any of the things that you used to do, then there is likely an underlying problem that your doctors should address.

The Energy Bank Account

Energy is like a bank account. This is true for everyone, not just cancer patients. You write a check against your energy account whenever you are active throughout the day. You might be doing something pleasant, such as hosting family for a dinner, going shopping, going to the movies, or spending time on your favorite hobby. It could be something less pleasant, such as a stressful meeting or a confrontation, cleaning the house (in my case), or doing anything that's boring but necessary. We all have those tasks in our lives.

When you are in treatment, the balance in your energy account is going to be lower than usual. So it's important to remember that everything you do expends precious energy. I urge patients to choose activities wisely and to make note of those times in the day when they usually have the most energy. Save those high-energy times to do the things that are most fulfilling. If you have a to-do list full of little chores that can be taken care of by someone else, now is your chance to delegate them all without guilt.

This may be a difficult adjustment at first. I have patients say to me that they would never dream of asking someone else to wash their car or mow the lawn or fold laundry. "I don't want to be a burden" is what they tell me. But if you spend a morning doing one of those things, you might not have energy left to spend time with your grandchildren or have coffee with friends.

Some people tell me that they absolutely love scrubbing the grout in the shower or that they find joy in washing the kitchen floor. I don't completely understand this, but if you get excited about dusting the house from top to bottom or detailing your car, then go for it.

Maximizing Your Energy

Running low on energy can be especially frustrating if you are the kind of person who likes to be up and around and doing things and talking to people. It will take time to learn how, but there are several ways you can maximize your energy:

Engage in daily exercise. This doesn't necessarily mean going to a gym or an exercise class. It can be something as simple as a walk every day. Get up and move around so that your muscles have a little bit of strength and stamina.

Get a good night's sleep. Pay attention to how much you are sleeping and what might be interfering with sleep.

Make plans to do something fun. This is an easy one. Spend time with people who make you feel good, and spend the most time doing things you absolutely love. Anticipating fun activities and people to see will give you extra energy during the day.

Causes of Episodic Fatigue

You already know that fatigue is a primary side effect of cancer treatment. Most patients feel this episodic fatigue in the 24 to 72 hours after an infusion or radiation treatment, and then it usually diminishes rapidly after those first few days. If your infusions have been scheduled for every two to three weeks, then you will have a week or two to feel more like your old self, but when these treatments occur weekly it can be kind of a grind. Just when you get your strength back, it's time to go back for another infusion. It can feel like a sort of catch-22. The cancer causes fatigue because it disrupts your body's normal functioning. And the treatment causes fatigue because it is attacking the cancer cells and also disrupting your body's normal functioning. But when the treatments work well, they will actually relieve the fatigue over time. When the tumors are controlled by the treatments, your energy level will likely improve.

Causes of Ongoing Fatigue

I always encourage patients to keep track of their energy levels over time. A family member or friend can help you remember and note how long it takes for your energy to rebound after a treatment and help track your sleep patterns and what times during the day you have the most energy. This is all good information for planning your time, but it also helps your medical team figure out what's going on if your fatigue suddenly gets more difficult to manage. Here we discuss some of the issues they will be thinking about or asking about if you have ongoing fatigue.

Have You Been on the Same Course of Treatment for Several Months?

Fatigue can accumulate over the course of treatment. As noted before, if you have had a string of infusions, your energy level may bounce back more slowly over time. A series of radiation treatments can also cause cumulative fatigue that lasts for a couple of weeks after the radiation ends. In patients who are on continuous pills or injections to treat their breast cancer, the fatigue may build up over time. Jenn has a patient who was initially feeling quite well on letrozole and abemaciclib. After several months, though, the patient felt more tired and said that the fatigue was stopping her from going out on her evening walks with her husband. She was even skipping her weekly brunch with her best girlfriends. Jenn reduced the dose of abemaciclib, and the patient's energy increased, which enabled her to return to these important activities.

Do You Have an Underlying Medical Condition?

Sudden fatigue can be related to medical conditions other than treatment. This might include low blood counts, which are discussed in chapter 5. The medical term for this is anemia. Your doctor will be following your blood counts closely and will be able to tell right away if this is a problem. If you do have anemia, you might need a blood transfusion. Fatigue can also be a sign of infection, and your doctor will want to rule that out.

Another common medical cause of fatigue is an underactive thyroid gland, also called hypothyroidism. If you already carry this diagnosis, sometimes such medications as iron or calcium supplements can interfere with the absorption of the thyroid replacement medication and make your hypothyroidism worse. There is an easy blood test to check for hypothyroidism so your doctors should rule that out as a treatable cause of severe fatigue.

Rarely patients can develop adrenal insufficiency if they have been on steroids for a long time. This is true even if you've been taking steroids intermittently with chemotherapy or with drugs like dexamethasone to prevent nausea. Your doctor can pick this up on some routine blood tests but may need to do additional tests to measure your adrenal function.

How Much Pain Are You Experiencing?

Patients with uncontrolled pain are often exhausted. Many of my patients tell me that they want to take fewer pain medications or want to stay at a lower dose of a medication, and then they find their pain to be more disruptive than they had anticipated. Experiencing pain all day or all night drains a great deal of energy. I often urge patients to manage their pain more aggressively if they are struggling with fatigue.

I have a patient named Diane who was struggling with back pain from bony metastases. Radiation helped, but she still had pain that was waking her up several times every night. Diane is usually a high-energy person, but lately, she was feeling like she had to drag herself through the day. She thought her fatigue was caused by her demanding job and busy family life, but she agreed that the disrupted sleep at night was becoming an issue. We discussed adding another pain medication at bedtime, and she tried taking a low dose of long-acting morphine along with the acetaminophen and ibuprofen she was already taking in the evening. Her husband attended the next visit and said that it was an amazing change. Diane was sleeping through the night and overall seemed more at ease, more like her energetic herself.

What Medications Are You Taking?

All kinds of medications can cause fatigue or sedation. Some meds, such as diphenhydramine (Benadryl), cause you to feel zonked, and you may already know that if the nurses have given this to you as part of your infusion. Patients taking Benadryl during infusions tend to doze off. Gabapentin (Neurontin), which can be used to treat neuropathic pain and hot flashes, can also cause sleepiness. Thankfully this effect tends to wear off for most people as the body gets used to medications, so your doctor may suspect that a newly prescribed medication could be causing your fatigue.

Opioids also cause you to feel sleepy. I know I just explained that not controlling your pain aggressively enough can leave you exhausted, and now I have to explain that taking opioids can also drain your energy, particularly during those first few days of taking the medication or the first few days of taking a higher dose. Yet opioids are a mainstay of cancer pain management, so you want to be communicating with your medical team about how well the pills are addressing the pain and how much they are affecting your level of fatigue. With some trial and error, you can find a dose and regimen of pain medication that relieves the discomfort and yet leaves you energetic enough to do the things you enjoy. If you are experiencing a lot of fatigue when you first start taking an opioid, you should know it won't last forever. You should feel more energy after two to three days as your body gets used to the medication.

Not all opioids are alike in their effects either. Short-acting opioids tend to cause more sedation than long-acting opioids. That makes sense because the medications tend to enter the bloodstream quickly, peak in potency after a couple of hours, and then wear off. That's why we use short-acting opioids for managing sudden pain, even though you are more likely to feel fatigue as the medication peaks. Long-acting opioids, by contrast, deliver a more consistent level of pain relief and therefore cause less sedation. So your doctor may want to switch you from multiple doses of short-acting opioid to a couple of doses of a long-acting medication if you have chronic pain and struggle with the fatigue that comes with the medication.

But even with long-acting opioids, I try to be mindful of a medicine's sedative effect when choosing a dosing schedule. For example, long-acting morphine can be dosed every 12 hours or every 8 hours. I occasionally find that some patients do better with smaller doses divided more frequently. For a patient who requires 120 milligrams of long-acting morphine in a day, I may dose it at 40 milligrams every 8 hours rather than 60 milligrams every 12, especially if a patient is feeling really fatigued. Many patients can get more consistent pain control and less sedation with these smaller, more frequent doses.

For patients on larger doses of opioids, fatigue from advanced cancer can be treated with methylphenidate (Ritalin). While there is no convincing data that methylphenidate can help with general cancer fatigue, this stimulant can often relieve sedation caused by higher doses of opioids.

Are You Eating and Drinking Enough?

Poor hydration and low food intake can contribute to fatigue. What's tricky with cancer is that some people may not feel like eating. Some loss of appetite is normal, and yet there can be a lot of friction within families around how much the patient is or is not eating. Instead of contributing to that friction, I tell patients to just do their best. If you find that you are losing weight, try eating multiple small meals throughout the day. (And see chapter 13 for more on this topic.)

A bigger concern is drinking enough fluids. You might want to keep track of how much water you drink throughout the day to make sure you are getting enough. If you become dehydrated during a difficult chemo regimen, you may need IV fluids intermittently to keep you hydrated and energized.

How Well Are You Sleeping at Night?

Lack of sleep can make fatigue worse. Unfortunately, a lot of patients struggle to get a good night's sleep. Uncontrolled pain can keep you awake. Certain medications, such as steroids (dexamethasone) used in many chemotherapy regimens, can cause insomnia. And so can anxious thoughts. Many people living with cancer find nighttime particularly difficult. The

222 Managing Symptoms and Side Effects

house is quiet, and there isn't anything to distract you from worrisome thoughts. All of your concerns can sneak up on you at three in the morning if you don't have any place to talk about these anxieties during the day. You may find that getting to sleep and staying asleep are challenging, and this will lead directly to daytime fatigue.

I always talk to my patients about what doctors call sleep hygiene, which is all of the habits that contribute to a good night's sleep. They include setting a regular bedtime and preparing for bed by avoiding the television and other screen time late at night. In fact, sleep experts suggest that you use your bed just for sleeping and sex, which may mean removing the television and finding a comfortable chair for nighttime reading. You will want to make sure that the bedroom is quiet, cool, and dark. An air conditioner or fan along with room-darkening shades can help with this.

I also advise patients to avoid naps when they can. On those days when you are wiped out from an infusion or fighting an infection, you can sleep as much as you need to, but on other days I urge people to limit themselves to one 20-minute nap. Set an alarm if you need to. Napping is a big contributor to poor sleep at night. If your body doesn't get a strong enough impulse that it needs sleep, you'll lie awake.

Many people ask whether they should be using medication such as zolpidem (Ambien), lorazepam (Ativan), trazodone, or melatonin to help with sleep. I think this is a reasonable way to treat insomnia. Some people use these medications only on days when they get steroids along with their chemotherapy, knowing that these steroids will keep them up. Other patients use a slightly higher dose of their regular pain medication at night (such as an opioid or gabapentin) because it helps with pain while also promoting sleep. I also sometimes prescribe other kinds of medications that can be sedating in low doses. These include mirtazapine (Remeron), which is an antidepressant, and olanzapine (Zyprexa), which in higher doses can treat thought disorders but works at low doses to treat anxiety and sleeplessness.

Are You Waking Early in the Morning Unable to Go Back to Sleep?

If sleeping is an issue, you might want to think more closely about emotional issues that can be disturbing your sleep. Early-morning wakening is a common sign of depression, and your clinician might suggest an antidepressant to help you regulate your mood. Some people don't like the idea of taking an antidepressant, or they think that they take quite enough medications and don't want any more. But I would encourage you to listen to a doctor who suggests that depression may be part of your clinical picture. We know that treating depression is critical to helping patients do as well as possible with their cancer treatment. Patients who are treated for depression do better than those who show signs of depression but refuse treatment.

How Are You Managing Your Anxiety?

Uncontrolled anxiety can be exhausting. Patients often come to me saying that their fatigue is worse lately, and when we talk more about what's going on, they reveal that they have new concerns about the future or about how treatment is going. Sometimes this new anxiety makes sleep elusive, sometimes it keeps you from exercising, and it can really interfere with doing the activities that you love to do, things that will give you energy. I can't stress enough how important it is to find a safe place to talk about any worries that you have. This is discussed more fully in chapter 17.

If anxiety is keeping you from sleeping, your doctor can prescribe some medications, such as lorazepam, to help you fall asleep. If this anxiety persists and you find that you need to use lorazepam frequently, your doctor may prescribe a longer-acting maintenance medication to treat anxiety (see chapter 17). You can also talk to a social worker or psychologist in the cancer center about using relaxation techniques to use when you feel panicked or overly worried.

Are You Exercising Regularly?

If you are spending large portions of the day in bed or on the couch, your body can become deconditioned, which means that your muscles aren't as strong. Then when you get up and move around, you feel more tired than usual. It's easy for people in treatment to get out of the habit of getting exercise, and then they are surprised when a couple of errands leaves them wiped out. There are going to be some days after an infusion when you really can't get out and exercise, but on those days when you feel a little stronger, you will want to stay active. Aerobic exercises are the most helpful, such as walking or riding a bike. Unless you have a health condition that precludes heart-pumping exercise (such as heart or lung issues), you should try to get about 150 minutes of aerobic exercise per week. You can discuss your exercise regimen with your medical team, but getting more exercise will improve your energy and your quality of life. This is all easier said than done, especially for people who weren't exercising prior to breast cancer. If you can get started on a regular exercise routine, you will be amazed at how much better you feel.

For people who have always exercised, this can also be an adjustment. My patient Esther had loved running all of her life and had run in a dozen marathons before her cancer diagnosis. When she was diagnosed with metastatic breast cancer, she was also diagnosed with a metastasis to her hip and underwent surgery and radiation. This really helped with the pain she had been having, but it left her unable to exercise while she recovered. Eventually, she began to feel a persistent fatigue and a kind of sadness that her body was losing some of its muscle tone. Over time, she began to walk and even jog with ease, but she didn't have the energy for long distance running. Instead, she started going to the gym to swim laps. Now she swims several times a week and her energy has rebounded. She said the swimming workouts make her feel better than running because she doesn't have to worry about the nagging knee problems that developed after decades of running. Now she can get back in shape without hurting her knees.

Medications for General Fatigue

While several medications work to treat the underlying causes of fatigue, such as pain or sleeplessness, there aren't a lot of medications that are known to specifically relieve the general fatigue that comes along with cancer and treatment. In some cases, I prescribe such stimulants as methylphenidate (Ritalin) or agents that promote wakefulness, such as modafinil. The data is not clear that any of these agents significantly improve fatigue, but when we have been through all the other strategies, it's worth a try.

I have worked with Ariella in my palliative care clinic for quite a long time. She is 57 and has a history of metastatic breast cancer that had been stable for years on hormonal treatments. After the cancer progressed, she started chemotherapy, which caused significant fatigue. She told me, "It's like the bed and the couch are sucking me in." Her most significant joy was playing with her 2-year-old twin grandsons who lived a few blocks away. However, in the last few months, she said she couldn't muster the energy to walk to their house. In fact, she didn't even want them to visit her while she was feeling so tired. This made her feel really sad. We talked through all the possible causes of the more persistent, progressive fatigue that she had been experiencing. Her blood counts were okay, so anemia was not an issue. She had a history of anxiety and depression that she felt was in good control on an antidepressant. She was hydrating, and her appetite was okay as well. She had always enjoyed walking and did feel that in the past this helped keep her energy level up. In this situation, it was completely reasonable to try out a medication to increase her energy.

A stimulant often works best if we suspect that the fatigue is caused by opioids, but I sometimes try this even when patients aren't on opioids. Methylphenidate is safe for most patients, so talk to your doctor. If you have a cardiac history, they may be more cautious in using it, as it can increase heart rate and blood pressure in some patients. Typically I would start with 5 milligrams at 8:00 a.m. and at noon. Nothing later than one or two o'clock in the afternoon, though, because taking a stimulant later in the day may interfere with sleep.

Methylphenidate is nice in that it is short acting and lasts about four hours. You don't have to take it every day. You can have it in your toolbox for those days you want an extra boost to feel more like yourself, like when you go out to lunch with friends. I always tell patients that this isn't going to give them enough energy to run a marathon, but it can offer enough of an energy boost to get out into the world again.

Ariella and I discussed a trial of methylphenidate each morning and noontime as needed to help boost her energy. When she saw me the next time in clinic, she came in with a big smile on her face, happy to report that she was back to walking and had seen her grandsons almost daily. She didn't feel she needed the noontime dose, so she was just taking it in the mornings.

Steroids, such as dexamethasone, can also increase energy. In fact, some of my patients love being given a steroid as part of their chemotherapy regimen because it gives them so much energy. Steroids are not a great long-term solution because they can cause such side effects as ulcers, thinning bones, muscle weakness, and fluid retention. Still, they can be helpful at a low dose given once in a while. Paula is another patient I work with in the palliative care clinic. She loved taking dexamethasone (Decadron) at the time of her chemotherapy treatments. When she was on a break from chemotherapy, she asked if I could prescribe her a few days of Decadron prior to her family's Christmas celebration. She wanted to feel a little boost in energy and appetite during her favorite family holiday. In consultation with her oncologist, I gave her a small supply of very low-dose steroid pills that she used during the holidays.

CHAPTER SEVENTEEN

Why Do People Keep Asking Whether I Am Depressed or Anxious?

It's normal to feel anxious or down while you are being treated for breast cancer. After all, you are dealing with treatments and side effects along with all of the normal pressures of work and family life. Your body may look or feel different. In addition, there may be uncertainty about how well treatments are working and what's going to happen in the future. Any one of these factors can trigger feelings of sadness and loss. While you might be suffering from a clinical depression or anxiety that requires treatment, you might not. In this chapter, I (Vicki) describe ways to distinguish between the common, normal reactions to your diagnosis and the signs and symptoms of depression or anxiety that need treatment.

Even if what you are experiencing is a normal adjustment to a new reality, that's not going to stop loved ones from asking you about your mood and insisting that you need help with your feelings if you won't talk about them. Many times in palliative care appointments, I hear from spouses or family members of patients who are determined that a loved one is depressed or needs a therapist or psychiatrist to deal with the diagnosis of cancer. I tell lots of patients and their families to move away from the notion that someone must be depressed just because they have cancer.

Cancer treatment is extremely challenging, both physically and emotionally. Even the process of diagnosis can trigger intense feelings of loss. It is normal to grieve the fact that life is not the same as it used to be. Feeling sad at times is completely normal, and no pill is going to take that away. What's not normal is the feeling that you are always down and that you can't find a way to enjoy your life. It is really important that we treat depression if it exists.

The Difference between Sadness and Depression

Depression is tricky to identify with cancer because so many of the symptoms that signal an acute depressive episode can be caused by the cancer itself. Think about it. The warning signs of depression include loss of sleep and appetite, weight loss, irritability, lack of energy, difficulty concentrating, feelings of helplessness or hopelessness, having negative thoughts, and a diminished interest in normal activities. This checklist is misleading for cancer patients because many of these symptoms can be caused by a cancer diagnosis, by the side effects of cancer, or by the side effects of treatment. And yet, between 15% and 25% of cancer patients do experience clinical depression while in treatment. And doctors know from research and experience that patients who are struggling with depression don't do as well in treatment, so it is crucial to diagnose and treat depression when it is present.

So how do we distinguish between the sadness and grief that's inherent in a big life change from a clinical depression that can affect your health? I always ask patients to talk about the things in their lives that they enjoy. If you were my patient, I would ask how you are spending your time. What do you enjoy doing, and are you taking the time to do it? Are you physically able to do it? Is there any part of your day or your week that you especially look forward to? In part, palliative care professionals ask about your favorite activities so we can help you brainstorm ways for you to live fully, even if some of your symptoms and side effects make these activities more challenging. But we also ask these questions to see how you are getting along generally. We want to know whether you are able to find activities to enjoy and to look forward to.

During my first visit with Imani, her husband Andre expressed his concern that Imani was depressed. He said, "We haven't gotten any good news lately, and she's been through so much. Can't you prescribe an antidepressant to help her?" Imani had initially been diagnosed and treated 10 years before with an early-stage breast cancer. She had been cancer free for six years before it returned. Treatment was going well for her until the tumor stopped responding to chemotherapy. Imani said she understood the cancer was becoming harder to treat, and she felt sad about the prognosis. She was also feeling more fatigue during the day.

When I asked Imani what things in life brought her the most joy, what she really loved doing, she lit up and said, "My girls, of course!" She recounted her recent dates with each of her four grown daughters, and their plans to go on a family vacation together. Imani also loved crafting and on the days when her energy was up, she told me that she was making each of her daughters a scrapbook filled with lots of memories. She said she felt grateful to be making these memories in the present, and while she hoped for more time, she said she was going to fill whatever time she had with quality family time.

It's normal for patients and their families to feel sad and overwhelmed. While Imani felt sad about the news of cancer progression on her most recent scans, she was not feeling depressed most of the time and was very much enjoying her favorite activities. Imani was actually coping well, using her time and energy for the things that really made her happiest. The more I talked to Andre, the more I realized that Imani's illness was having a big impact on his life. I began to wonder whether he would benefit from a place to talk through his worries about the future. It's easy to underestimate how much strain spouses and family members are working under. Sometimes the person demanding therapy for the patient is the one in need of a little extra support. In palliative care, we know that we need to address the needs of the family so that the patient can do as well as possible.

Jill expressed a similar concern about her mother, Marsha, who had a prognosis similar to Imani. Although Marsha had been coping well with her diagnosis and treatment, Jill said that her mood had been getting worse over time. Marsha had been crying a lot at home and wasn't attending her weekly dates with her friends. She was an avid golfer and reader, but she had not gone golfing or read a book in months. When I asked Marsha how she felt, she admitted to feeling sad on most days and that even when her energy level was high, she did not feel motivated or interested in seeing her friends or even getting out of the house. I was much more worried that this was a true depression and not just sadness about the cancer.

When thinking about mood, doctors don't worry about the fact that you have down days. Everyone does. We worry instead about whether your mood can rebound. When I suspect a clinical depression, I do urge patients to seek treatment, which can be in the form of talk therapy or medication. In the meantime, the first step in feeling better is making sure that your cancer and/or cancer therapy symptoms and side effects are under control.

Uncontrolled Symptoms Affect Mood

Almost any physical symptom can affect your mood. You might feel that you are being strong in not taking much pain medication, for example, but then you find that the discomfort is sapping your energy or distracting you from doing the simplest activities, such as watching a movie or taking a walk. The same is true with nausea, bowel trouble, insomnia, difficulty eating, or anxiety. Over time, these side effects of treatment can chip away at your resolve, even if you don't think of them as big problems individually. This is especially true if you haven't felt comfortable talking about them with your oncologist. A terrific benefit of working with palliative care is that we can take the time to ask lots of questions about how you are getting along day to day and find ways to get these problems under control.

I once had a patient struggling with severe diarrhea, which was a side effect of her chemotherapy regimen. She hadn't talked much to her oncologist about how bad the diarrhea really was. She was embarrassed to talk about it in detail, which is understandable. Over time, she became fearful of leaving the house because she was afraid that she wouldn't be able to find a bathroom in time. Her life became smaller and smaller until she was showing signs of depression. Once she was able to describe the problem to me, I devised a plan to lessen the impact of the diarrhea in her life. We couldn't eliminate it, but we got her to the point where she could go shopping again and she could go out with her family and visit her friends. Her mood improved dramatically.

When Can Anxiety or Depression Emerge?

Anxiety and depression can surface at any point in time, so it's something your doctors and nurses will ask you about frequently. That said, it is common to feel anxious or depressed soon after the diagnosis and when you start cancer treatments. You can even experience some difficult emotions when the treatment is going well.

People who are undergoing curative treatments may actually start to experience these symptoms after treatment ends. Without the regularly scheduled lab draws, visits, nursing checks, infusions, and frequent visits, sometimes there is more time to think about the cancer diagnosis and to cope with what has just happened. For others, the time of year when the diagnosis happened may trigger feelings of depression and anxiety that are transient. Jenn has a patient who is several years out from her breast cancer treatment who experiences intense anxiety in the weeks before her yearly mammograms and visits. It's normal for any person with a history of breast cancer to experience some anxiety before a mammogram; but for this patient, the fear of recurrence was dominating her life in those weeks before her mammograms. It was impairing her ability to work, sleep, and be present with her family. She is now seeing a therapist a few weeks prior to her yearly mammogram. This has really helped her to diminish the anxiety she had been experiencing.

You may not expect this, but people who remain cancer-free years beyond their diagnosis can still experience high rates of anxiety. If you feel that the fear of recurrence is interfering with your quality of life, you may want to seek out additional supports like connecting with a therapist and discuss with your team any symptoms of anxiety or depression that you may be experiencing. During your visits, your team will ask you about your mood so that they can help you feel better.

Practical Talk Therapy

Perhaps you've tried talk therapy in the past and benefitted from it, or perhaps you are resistant to the idea of talking to a psychologist or social worker about your emotions. Even if you've never tried therapy before, it can really help you cope with the strong emotions that come with a cancer diagnosis. You already know that having cancer isn't like having other problems. It's a different beast entirely, one that complicates all of the relationships in your life, and yet there are many feelings and frustrations that you share with other cancer patients. It's tempting to think that these issues are too big to talk about or that talking alone won't help. But talk therapy can help, particularly if it comes with practical advice and strategies for coping. Research conducted at Mass General has found that patients who engage with a palliative care professional in the early months after diagnosis experienced a 50% lower rate of depression compared to other patients. We didn't prescribe more antidepressants. Instead, we gave patients a place to discuss their worries and find things to hope for, and we helped them plan for the future.

I've found that helping patients focus on the future is vital. You may need help finding something to look forward to, something to do that is immersive and meaningful. You want to stay engaged in life, and that can be harder at various points in the process. I find that many patients with serious cancers are afraid to just live. I don't know why, but perhaps it's because everything seems so uncertain. So I try to ask people, "What do you want to do next?" If the answer is a trip to the Grand Canyon with family, I can say, "Great. Let's get your symptoms under control, do some practical planning to make sure you are feeling your best, and buy some travel insurance in case you feel crummy." Patients often tell me that they need to stay optimistic while dealing with cancer, and by that they seem to mean that they have to stay focused on beating the cancer. Instead, I urge people to feel optimistic about enjoying life right now. It's okay to let go and let the clinical team worry about how the treatment is working. One patient said to me, "So let me get this straight. You are going to tell me when I should be more worried about my cancer, and in the meantime, I can just do my thing?" Yes, I said. To which she replied, "That sounds good to me."

Talk therapy can help you focus on your goals and your identity outside of cancer treatment. Most people have some sense of what brings their life purpose. It may be a fulfilling career, relationships with family and friends, or religion. When cancer drops into your life, that sense of purpose may get distorted or lost. Some patients feel that they are so often at the cancer center or getting tests, scans, seeing doctors, or getting treatments that their identity gets wrapped up in the cancer diagnosis. Some people have to leave their jobs; others may feel frustrated that they don't have the energy or time to do the things they enjoy doing or quality time with their loved ones. I was caring for a teacher who loved nothing more than sharing her passion for physics with her middle-schoolers. On weekly chemotherapy, she felt a lot of fatigue and had to take a leave of absence from work. She really struggled with the feeling that she had lost her sense of purpose. We talked about some practical strategies to time her chemotherapy on Fridays rather than Mondays, and about options to get her back to doing what she loved. She's now working part time tutoring science several days a week, and she finds this has restored some of her sense of identity and meaning as a teacher.

You do want to take some care in finding a therapist who has experience working with cancer patients. If you have the chance to engage with a palliative care professional, you know that this person has a lot of experience helping patients manage symptoms and side effects of cancer and can give solid advice about dealing with it emotionally. You can also ask someone at the hospital or cancer clinic to recommend other therapists with experience treating people who have cancer and all of the unknowns that come with the diagnosis. Where a social worker or traditional psychologist can provide an incredibly helpful space to talk through issues more indirectly related to your diagnosis (e.g, if you need to talk about getting your ex-husband to be more supportive of your teenage children), you want to work with someone who understands the unique needs of cancer patients when seeking help with your own anxiety or depression.

Medications

If talking isn't enough, you might consider medication to relieve depression. Some patients tell me that they don't want to take another medication or that they believe that they shouldn't have to take medication for depression. I always say that you are not being a wimp by addressing one of your symptoms. Does it make sense to be going through cancer treatment when you are not at the top of your game? Depression needs to be treated if it affects your life.

I also remind patients that there are lots of options for antidepressants (table 17.1) and that these pills are very well tolerated, which means that they bring few side effects. They also work fairly quickly, within two to four weeks, and can have other benefits for cancer patients. For example, some antidepressants increase appetite or help with sleep. Many antidepressants can also help with hot flashes, which is a common side effect of hormonal therapies and menopause.

Selective serotonin reuptake inhibitors (commonly known as SSRIs), such as citalopram (Celexa), escitalopram (Lexapro), and sertraline (Zoloft), are effective and have few side effects. Your doctor will likely prescribe the starting dose, and if you are not feeling better, this dose can be increased. And if the first medication prescribed by your team isn't effective, you have other options. Or if you were on an antidepressant in the past that really helped, be sure to let your doctor know. Often if you felt better on a medication in the past, the odds are that it will help again.

Once you're underway with treatment, continue to check in with your doctor about how you are feeling. It's important to keep depression in check.

Anxiety

Cancer treatment brings a lot of anxiety into your life. Of course it does. Who wouldn't be anxious before getting the results from a test that your doctor ordered? Who doesn't worry about the possibility that the treatment won't work as well as everyone hopes? For some women, they feel they are always waiting for the other shoe to drop. Even if they are feeling well and things are going smoothly from their doctor's perspective, they worry about what's to come.

Table 17.1. Common medications used to treat depression

Class	Common drugs in the class	Side effect profile
SSRI (selective serotonin reuptake inhibitor)	Fluoxetine (Prozac), sertraline (Zoloft), citalopram (Celexa), escitalopram (Lexapro), paroxetine (Paxil)	Generally very well tolerated. Some people can experience dry mouth, diarrhea, and sexual dysfunction. Paroxetine, in particular, interacts with many medications prescribed for cancer patients for nausea, etc., so we try to avoid it.
SNRI (serotonin-norepinephrine reuptake inhibitor)	Duloxetine (Cymbalta), venlafaxine (Effexor XR)	Well tolerated for patients who are not responding to an SSRI. Duloxetine has been shown to help with neuropathic pain.
NDRI (norepinephrine-dopamine reuptake inhibitor)	Buproprion (Wellbutrin)	Buproprion is a helpful medication for patients who have fatigue as a big part of their depressive symptoms. Well tolerated, few to no sexual side effects. Can cause headache, dry mouth, nausea, and constipation.
Atypical	Mirtazapine (Remeron)	Sedating, usually given at bedtime to help with sleep. Can also help with appetite.
Tricyclic antidepressants	Nortriptyline (Pamelor), amitriptyline (Elavil), doxepin	May be used in low doses to help with pain or sleep. Used to treat depression only if other antidepressants have not worked. In the higher doses used to treat depression, we see dry mouth and constipation.
Neuroleptics	Olanzapine (Zyprexa), quetiapine (Seroquel)	May be used to augment the effect of an SSRI or other antidepressant. Olanzapine, in particular, is being used more frequently as an antinausea medication, appetite stimulant, antianxiety medication, and sleep aid.

It's normal to feel anxious about the future. Sometimes the anxiety is going to make it more difficult to concentrate, more difficult to fall asleep at night, or more difficult to enjoy some of the ordinary pleasures in life. Some people feel this very real anxiety and then are able to let it go or set it aside for a little while. Maybe they find an engrossing activity or a mindless distraction. Maybe they engage in meditation or praycr. Maybe they find a place to talk about worries in a way that lessens their impact.

Other people really struggle with anxiety to the point where it affects their day-to-day lives. If you have struggled with anxiety in the past, you may find cancer treatment makes this anxiety worse. Tell your doctor if your anxiety is keeping you from sleeping or eating or functioning in your life. Feeling overwhelmed by anxiety is not a failure on your part. I consider anxiety to be a side effect of cancer, and it should be treated as such. The goal is to prevent anxiety from adversely affecting your life each day. You can try some of the coping strategies in chapter 6, or you can try talk therapy, and if you need help for acute anxiety or panic, there are several medications that can help. You can't take all the worries away, but you can lessen them with help.

The Negative Power of Positive Thinking

Many people feel tempted to cope with anxiety by pretending they don't feel it. I find this particularly true for people who say that positive thinking is the key to success in everything. General optimism in life can be incredibly powerful because it helps you take on tough challenges and try new things. Cancer is a different kind of challenge, though, because there are so many aspects you can't control. You can't control the biology of your tumor, and you can't control how effective treatment is going to be.

Some patients don't want to ever acknowledge that there are things they can't control about their cancer. They feel that this vulnerability will be too overwhelming. Instead, they tell themselves over and over again that they need to stay positive all the time, every minute. Friends and family members can feed this thinking, too, by telling you that you are strong, that you are a warrior, and that you are going to beat this. There is nothing wrong with saying these things or feeling them, but this kind of relentless optimism can actually create anxiety.

I had a patient recently, Julie, who was having a lot of trouble sleeping. She had trouble falling asleep at night and then would wake up at two or three in the morning with her mind racing. I asked her what she was thinking about when she couldn't sleep, but she didn't want to tell me at first. Finally, she admitted that she was worrying about what would happen if her cancer got worse. She worried about her husband and how he would care for her if she were really sick, and how she would be letting him down if she didn't get better. Then she sat up straighter and said, "But I can't think like that. I have to stay positive." She wasn't really talking to me at that point. She was lecturing herself. She also said that if she didn't stay optimistic, she was inviting her cancer to grow.

I hear this a lot, and I know that optimism can be a useful tool to help you cope with a crummy situation. But it's not healthy to police your thoughts all the time or to completely deny the normal fears and negative thoughts that come with a serious diagnosis. Negative thoughts can't be pushed aside forever. If you deny them, they pop up when you least expect them, usually in the middle of the night. In palliative care, we encourage people to talk about their worries, to talk about what might happen if the cancer gets worse, even if they can only do so for a few minutes at a time. We do this because it is another great tool for coping. By acknowledging your worries, they lessen their control over you.

I worked with Julie on this, asking the questions that I ask all of my patients:

What has your oncologist said about what might happen in the future?

When you think about the future, what do you think about?

What do you worry might happen?

What if one of the things you worry about did happen? What would that be like?

Can we think of some strategies for how you would cope with this if it did happen?

How can your family get support if something like this did happen?

Allowing yourself to talk about what might happen and what you worry about doesn't invite your cancer to get worse. It's just another conversation that falls under the heading "What If." And while you can have these conversations with a palliative care professional, you can also have them with a close friend or family member, or a therapist experienced with cancer treatment.

At first it was difficult for Julie to admit to the things that she worried most about. These conversations take practice. Over time she found that she could describe more of her concerns about the future. She wondered how much longer she could work. She worried that if she stopped working, she wouldn't be able to afford college for her kids. She worried about who would care for her aging mother. She wondered aloud if she could really die from her cancer. These are enormous concerns, and yet she hadn't talked to anyone about them. Her need to stay positive had actually isolated her from her family and prevented her from thinking of any practical solutions.

We talked about the possibility of her working reduced hours or going on short-term disability so that she could focus on her health. We talked about ways for her to get more support for her mother. I also referred her to a social worker in the cancer center so that she would have more help addressing these issues. After every one of our conversations, Julie told me that she still wanted to be positive about her prognosis, and that's great. Talking about your worries doesn't mean that you have to think about them all of the time. Giving them a little airtime allows you feel less alone and gives you more energy to focus on your health and your immediate goals.

Using the Box

Julie had other concerns about her diagnosis and what the future would look like. It was harder for her to talk about these subjects than it was for her to talk about the practical problems of work and money. So I introduced her to the idea of the box (also described in chapter 6). I told her that we could tackle one subject at a time and only for as long as she wanted to talk, and the rest of it could stay in the imaginary box until she was ready. She had complete control. She would say, "Let's open the box for a minute." And then she would tell me one of her concerns, which were all of the normal worries. What if the next scan isn't good news? What if I get sick? What if my husband has to care for me? What if that's really hard for him? What if it's too hard for my kids to see me getting worse? What if I die? What will happen to my family?

These concerns were also causing enormous anxiety, and pretending they didn't exist wasn't working for her. We would pick one of these questions and talk about it for as long as she wanted, sometimes only a few minutes. When she felt that we had talked long enough or when she was feeling that the topic was too much, she would say, "I think it's time to close the box." At that point, we would stop. We completely compartmentalized these conversations, and that gave her the confidence to talk about what was bothering her most without the fear of being overwhelmed. Gradually, she was able to make practical plans for what might happen if her cancer got worse and how she and her family could better cope. Eventually she found herself feeling much more like the capable, competent person she had always been.

Many of my patients have become very comfortable using the box technique. Some of these women have partners or family members who are so focused on the positive that they have a tough time listening to any talk about practical concerns. Alma has metastatic breast cancer that has been stable for a while. She is also a mother of three teenagers. Even though she feels well, she has tried to engage her partner, Erik, in drawing up a will and considering what things they would want for their children in the long term. He keeps saying, "You just have to stay positive. You're going to be fine." Alma knows he is trying to be helpful, but this approach does not alleviate her anxiety about their kids or what the future might bring for their family. I invited her to have Erik join us for a visit so that I could help facilitate some of these discussions. She has also started to confide in one of her closest friends, and it's been helpful for her to have this additional source of support.

Medication for Anxiety

Although talking about anxieties can help relieve them, you might have acute episodes of anxiety or panic or ongoing difficulty sleeping that might require medication. In some instances, anxiety feels like a giant wave that can knock you over. Antianxiety medication doesn't take the worries away, but it can help you to keep standing when the wave hits. As with depression, you want to treat anxiety by also making sure that your other cancer-related symptoms and side effects are under control.

I met Yvette soon after her diagnosis of an early-stage breast cancer. She was working full-time as a bartender and at each chemotherapy visit, she would bring in a different group of very devoted friends who would also check in on her regularly at home. She had a great support system and a busy life and did great throughout her chemotherapy and year of trastuzumab (Herceptin). A couple of months after she finished trastuzumab, however, Yvette told me that she was feeling a lot of anxiety. She said that there had been a comfort to her routine of coming to the clinic for labs, appointments, and infusions. When she needed less frequent visits, she felt a little lost. At night, her mind raced and became flooded with lots of thoughts about everything from mundane work tasks to worries about death and dying. She was also having difficulty concentrating at work and was irritable with her family and friends. Although she was open to seeing a therapist, she wanted to hold off on starting medications at first. Her therapist gave her some techniques to address the racing thoughts at night, which allowed her to get more rest, but anxiety was still a problem for her during the day.

Similar to the effect on depression, medications such as SSRIs can be very helpful for this kind of anxiety. Your doctor may start you on a low dose that may need to be increased if you are not feeling better over time. Doctors also sometimes prescribe short-acting antianxiety medications, such as lorazepam (Ativan), for the first two to four weeks while waiting for the SSRI to start working. Sometimes the clinical team worries that combining lorazepam and pain medications can cause confusion. In this situation, I sometimes suggest low doses of a different medication, such as olanzapine (Zyprexa). This kind of medication works more quickly than an SSRI and treats confusion instead of causing it. It is a terrific medication for intense anxiety.

I started Yvette on lorazepam and an SSRI, and her anxiety improved a great deal. She told me that she was pleasantly surprised by the results, saying, "I feel like myself again." After almost a year, Yvette decided to go off the medication, and she is still feeling great off the SSRI.

Integrative Therapies to Reduce Depression and Anxiety

People often ask me what other therapies they can use in order to reduce depression, anxiety, or stress. The Society for Integrative Oncology reviewed published studies to find the most effective integrative therapies during and after breast cancer treatment. Meditation has the most robust evidence for improving mood disturbance and depressive symptoms and reducing anxiety. There is good evidence as well to support the use of relaxation in people who are experiencing depressive symptoms.

Therapists can help teach relaxation techniques, and there are numerous telephone and tablet apps that can guide you through meditation and relaxation techniques.

Music therapy and yoga are also both recommended for alleviating depression and anxiety. A lot of people like the flexibility of being able to add one or several of these interventions into their life since they really may help and don't involve pills or side effects.

CHAPTER EIGHTEEN

How Does Cancer Affect My Brain?

Many people worry that the treatments they receive for breast cancer will affect their thinking. Most patients have heard of "chemo brain," which is a term the medical community has given to the very common complaint from individuals that their cognitive function isn't the same when they are undergoing cancer treatment, particularly chemotherapy. But women who take hormonal therapies also report these effects. People report that their thinking isn't as sharp or that they can't complete a brainteaser or crossword puzzle as easily. They can't multitask the way they used to or concentrate on complicated tasks at work. There are many causes for these complaints, and only sometimes do they involve breast cancer therapies. Cancer treatment brings a lot of stressors, including fatigue, anxiety, multiple medications, and a host of medical details to track. Any one of these factors can affect your ability to carry out complex tasks. Radiation to the brain can also cause cognitive impairment.

People are often reluctant to admit to confusion, even to a doctor, but when you do speak up, the doctor can begin to look for some of the known causes and may be able to help. Many times, your doctor will be able to tease out the problem and isolate a medication or other part of treatment that may be contributing to the problem. But doctors take complaints about brain function seriously because once in a while this can indicate that something more urgent is happening. This chapter describes the most common causes for cognitive impairment and what will happen if the cancer is directly affecting your brain.

What Is Chemo Brain Exactly?

Chemo brain describes a patient's experience of mental fogginess during and after cancer treatments. It is a kind of catch-all term to refer to cognitive changes attributable to cancer therapies, which may include chemotherapy, hormonal therapy, and even surgery and radiation. People often report difficulties with memory, focus, attention, problems finding words, and multitasking. If you are experiencing these symptoms, your doctor will examine you to make sure that your symptoms are not related to progressive cancer. Your doctor will also want to look for potentially reversible factors that might be contributing, such as depression, fatigue, pain, sleep disturbances, and medications. Some institutions have a specialized team who are trained in assessing cognitive function with a battery of tests called neuropsychiatric testing.

It's often helpful to know that you are experiencing something that really might be related to your treatments and that this will likely improve after your treatment ends. For most people treated with chemotherapy for an early-stage breast cancer, cognitive dysfunction does not worsen over time, and many experience improvement within a year after completing chemotherapy. One of my patients with early-stage breast cancer told me that after she read some information online about chemo brain, she actually felt better knowing that she was not alone in her experience and that she would likely get better over time.

If you do experience thinking and memory problems while in treatment, you can use several strategies to help you stay oriented in the short term. We usually recommend using planners, lists, smartphone reminders, and alarms to help keep you on track. Experts also recommend exercise to improve focus, as well as relaxation techniques, meditation, and yoga to help with stress. For some, cognitive rehabilitation may include occupational therapy, speech therapy, and psychotherapy.

What Your Doctor Will Ask

When you are describing difficulties with thinking or confusion or your worries about your brain to your clinical team, they will try to figure out whether this could be caused by the side effects of treatment or whether the cancer itself is directly affecting your brain function. Your medical team will be wondering about a host of possible triggers, and it can take time to sort them all out.

I (Jenn) have a patient with an estrogen-positive breast cancer that has spread to her bones. Bonnie is a corporate attorney who describes herself as a super type-A-plus person who works long hours during the week. On the weekends, she takes flying lessons in a small Cessna. She has been doing great on hormonal therapy and her most recent CT scans and bone scans showed stability in the cancer. When she came to see me for a routine visit and described how long it was taking her to complete regular responsibilities at work and how hard it was to stay on task, I knew that this didn't sound like Bonnie.

To tease out the problem, I asked her all of the questions doctors usually pose in this situation:

Do you also have headaches?

Do you have any specific difficulties with movement or walking?

Do you have difficulty with speaking or seeing things?

Has anyone ever said they thought you were confused?

Do you ever wonder whether you have lost consciousness?

Has a friend or family member thought that you've lost consciousness?

She said no to all of these questions, but I still ordered an MRI to make sure she had no brain metastases. When the MRI came back clear, we could focus on what other things might be causing her problem. She admitted that she had been working more overtime than usual on a complex case and had been getting far less sleep. Her primary care doctor had prescribed lorazepam (Ativan, a benzodiazepine that relieves anxiety) to help her get to sleep at night. Fatigue, stress, and medications are very common causes of cognitive impairment, and any one of these factors might have been playing on role in why Bonnie felt less sharp than usual.

Bonnie admitted that she had been using the lorazepam during the day as well to help with some of the stress at work. Lorazepam is a drug that can certainly interfere with short-term memory. She decided to limit her use of this drug to a single dose at bedtime. In addition, she started working with a therapist who could give her other stress reduction techniques, including mindfulness work. She also started exercising, which is another way to reduce stress, improve focus, and promote better sleep. We also worked on strategies to help her stay on task and improve her memory, including list-making and cognitive exercises.

In some cases, we offer methylphenidate as well to stimulate the ability to concentrate. This is more common for those people faced with the sedation and cognitive side effects from opioids in the setting of advanced cancer.

Other Causes of Cognitive Impairment

Breast cancer therapies can have some effect on thinking, but there are also many other things you go through in treatment that can disrupt your thinking:

- Medications, particularly pain medications and benzodiazepines (including antianxiety medications, such as lorazepam). Antinausea medications can also be a culprit.

- Radiation therapy to the brain can cause difficulties in attention, short-term memory, and processing.

- Anxiety and lack of sleep can cause short-term memory difficulties. So can depression.

- Cancer spreading to the brain can cause some of these issues, as well.

Delirium

Some patients experience a temporary but noticeable state of confusion called delirium. It has many potential causes, including something as benign as medication or as easily treatable as a developing infection. But it can also be a sign of a new brain lesion (that is, tumor), a seizure, or a stroke.

I recently admitted one of my colleague's patients to the hospital. Sally has metastatic breast cancer, and her husband became concerned when she woke in the middle of the night and got dressed for work. She seemed to be in a haze, and when her husband asked her what she was doing, she said, "I have to go to work." He couldn't convince her otherwise. He got dressed and drove her to the hospital, which was the right thing to do.

If a patient experiences delirium, doctors consider this an emergency unless the cause is obvious and reversible. For example, if the patient has taken too much lorazepam or too much of an opioid, they may experience several hours of confusion. Many times the cause isn't obvious, and the patient needs to come to the hospital to go through an evaluation. In the hospital, doctors will take a careful history of events, do a physical exam, and draw blood. The goal is rule out all the possible causes of delirium. If nothing obvious emerges, doctors usually suggest an MRI and may consult with neurologists to figure out what's going on.

In Sally's case, the original work-up revealed no reason for her confusion. She fell asleep waiting for a bed in the hospital, and when she woke she felt completely normal and showed no signs of confusion. I sat down with her and went over the events of the previous day. Sally remembered dropping her pills on the ground. She thought that she had put all the pills back in their correct bottles but wasn't sure. Her husband produced her pill bottles (it's always good to bring those to the hospital in this kind of emergency). When we looked, we realized that she had mixed up a couple of the pills. As a result, she had taken three times the amount of lorazepam that was prescribed. Because she had tumors in her liver, her body had trouble processing the extra medication, and this had been the cause of her delirium.

Spacing Out

In some cases, delirium or confusion can arise from a more serious cause. My patient Natasha has metastatic breast cancer and was doing well on chemotherapy. She was working part time and enjoying every weekend with her grandchildren at her daughter's pool. One day, her daughter called me to report that Natasha was sitting by the pool the day before and staring off into space. She wouldn't respond to any questions for a minute or so. Then she would rouse herself and begin a new conversation, seemingly unaware that she'd missed everything that had been said to her. It wasn't clear to me what might be causing this to happen. I told Natasha's daughter that it could be anything, including dehydration, an infection, or something more serious related to the cancer. Natasha came to the emergency room for an evaluation and scans. Brain imaging unfortunately showed new metastases. These episodes of spacing out had been miniseizures. I got her started right away on antiseizure medication to stop the episodes and then got her set up for radiation therapy to help treat the metastases.

What If My Cancer Goes to My Brain?

Women with metastatic breast cancer frequently worry about the prospect of their cancer metastasizing to the brain the way that it does to the liver or to any other part of the body. Any breast cancer can metastasize to the brain, but certain types of breast cancer have an increased tendency to do this, including triple-negative and HER2-positive breast cancers. Patients who experience the sudden onset of headaches, confusion, or difficulty speaking or moving may be showing signs of brain metastases. Patients who complain of these symptoms will often undergo an MRI of the brain to determine whether this is the case. MRIs are better than CT scans at evaluating the brain.

I was caring for Crystal, a woman in her midfifties who had been incredibly healthy until she was diagnosed with triple-negative breast cancer that had spread to her liver and lungs. She was one of those patients who rarely reported any concerns about side effects. So when she told me that she had been experiencing some weakness and numbness in her right leg, I was concerned. Crystal told me that she thought she had simply pulled a muscle or two during a tennis game over the weekend. I checked in with her oncologist who agreed that she should get a brain MRI. Unfortunately, the MRI showed two brain metastases that were causing some swelling.

Crystal was devastated, as most people are when they first hear that their cancer has spread to the brain. This news can feel overwhelming, but your medical team will put together a plan to address it. Your oncologist will tell you that controlling the disease in the brain will become the primary focus. Sometimes you will be able to continue taking anti-cancer medication that is controlling the cancer in the rest of your body, but sometimes you will need to put that on hold.

Depending on the size, location, and number of metastases involved, your oncologist may consult with neurosurgeons to see whether they can be removed. Your doctor will also be considering what kind of symptoms you have because of the brain lesions. Radiation oncologists will also weigh in to determine whether the lesions should be irradiated, and if so, how. Sometimes surgeons will want to operate even when they know they can't remove all of the tumors that are causing inflammation in the brain tissue. Remember that the skull is like a wooden box that encases the brain, and if there is a large metastasis that is causing symptoms, your medical team may decide to remove some part of the cancer to relieve the swelling. Doctors might recommend stereotactic radiosurgery (in which a high dose of radiation is delivered to the small area of the cancer nodule), proton beam radiotherapy, or even operative surgery. In some cases, the whole brain needs to be treated with radiation therapy, which may require that you stop the other anti-cancer treatments that you are using.

If you have brain metastases, your doctor may also prescribe steroids, such as dexamethasone, to keep the swelling at a minimum. These drugs can keep your brain functioning well, and sometimes doctors tell patients that they should continue to take them to prevent further swelling and inflammation that the cancer is causing in the brain. That said, some patients don't like taking steroids because of the potential for side effects. Over the course of several weeks, steroids can cause your face to swell. You might gain weight, you can develop high blood sugar, and your muscles can weaken. Your team will provide guidance on whether you might be able to decrease the dose of steroids and if you can eventually stop taking them.

In Crystal's case, she was admitted to the hospital and started on steroids, which reduced the inflammation in her brain and eased some of the numbness she had been feeling in her right leg. The neurosurgery and radiation oncology teams met during her hospitalization and decided that the best treatment would be stereotactic radiosurgery to both of the brain lesions. This can deliver precise doses of radiation and can be very effective for small brain lesions.

Her oncologist also ordered new CT scans to see if the cancer was spreading in the rest of her body. These scans showed that the cancer was still responding well to the chemotherapy and was stable in the rest of her body. This is not unusual. One unfortunate limitation of many cancer therapies is that they work less well in the brain. Your body is equipped with something called the blood-brain barrier. It works great to keep toxins, including infections, out of your brain even if they are circulating in your system. But this barrier also keeps many cancer therapies from getting to your brain and killing the cancer cells there. That's why someone like Crystal can have a great result from chemotherapy in her body, and yet the lesions are freer to grow in her brain.

The Role of Rehab

When patients have cancer in the brain, they can sometimes suffer the neurologic damage that is often associated with strokes. They may have balance issues or difficulty speaking and understanding language. When someone has a stroke and is otherwise doing pretty well, doctors suggest physical therapy and occupational therapy as a way to help people regain the skills they may have lost. It's always an option to get these therapies to help you live better and feel better.

In the setting of metastatic cancer, sometimes patients have trouble scheduling these other therapies while receiving intensive treatments for the cancer itself. In some cases, by the time the cancer spreads to the brain, the patient is already exhausted from treatment and from the tumor burden, meaning the amount of cancer in the body. Some patients say to their doctors that they don't really want to spend two to four weeks in a rehab facility practicing walking or learning an exercise regimen because they would rather be at home. Your medical team should understand this request. Your doctors should try to balance this work to regain neurologic function with all of the other demands on you as a patient.

PART THREE

Dealing with Progressing Cancer

CHAPTER NINETEEN

They Tell Me the Cancer is Progressing

If your cancer isn't curable, there will be a point at which the cancer grows despite treatment and begins to spread. You may decide to read this chapter because scans are showing that the primary tumor has grown or that new tumors have appeared in other parts of your body. If you have been hospitalized for side effects related to the cancer, such as pain or an infection, your doctor may have ordered new scans to see whether these have been caused by the spread of cancer. In some cases, patients have had a great response from targeted therapies or standard chemotherapy, and then suddenly they become ill with a complication from the cancer.

When your doctor says that the cancer is progressing despite treatment, they are telling you that you are, in fact, at a different phase of treatment. This can be hard to accept. Many patients say that they needed weeks or even months to understand fully that their cancer was advancing, and patients often ask us what it means to have advancing cancer. I (Jenn) say that up to now your medical team has been working to minimize the symptoms and side effects of treatment, but in the future we will be working with you to minimize the side effects of the cancer itself. Some people may experience more symptoms from cancer as it progresses, and your team will recommend treatments to help minimize symptoms like pain and shortness of breath. Not everyone will have these symptoms. Some people have few side effects of advancing cancer except for an increase in fatigue and weight loss.

Some women with metastatic breast cancer can be on one treatment after another, sometimes for months or years at a time. We always start with treatments that are likely to provide the best shot at controlling the cancer for the longest time. The tumor will eventually progress despite treatment, and there will be a discussion about whether there is another effective treatment to switch to. With each subsequent line of therapy there may be less of a response or a response for a shorter period of time. At some point, the treatments become less effective, and the body may be too weak for more treatment. For those women who have been living with metastatic breast cancer for a long time, sometimes years, this can be especially confusing because they are used to having many treatment options that can control the cancer. It is hard to hear that the risks and burdens of more treatment may outweigh the benefits.

When a cancer shows that it can grow through the first-line treatment (meaning the first treatment that you try), it may mean that changing to another regimen will control the cancer nearly as well as the first. However, it may mean that the cancer has acquired the ability to grow through second-, third-, and fourth-line treatments. Over the years, patients have often told us that they get frustrated with their doctors at this point because the oncologists become more guarded when talking about prognosis. We've all had patients for whom a change in therapy was a minor bump in the road and the next round of chemotherapy got the cancer under control for a long time. But we've also had patients where progressive cancer can't be controlled by more treatment. People think that we can tell which ones will be which. The truth is that we can't know, so there is some uncertainty each time we have to change treatment because the cancer is worsening.

Entering a New Phase

Hearing that you are in a new phase of treatment can make you feel vulnerable all over again. Many patients say that learning the primary tumor is growing or that new metastases have become visible is a shock similar to the one they felt when they were first diagnosed. In the next chapter, Vicki will talk about how to cope in this new phase, how to develop a good awareness of the likely course and outcome of your disease, and what to hope for when you can't hope for a cure. Getting oriented in this new reality takes time, and you need to be patient with yourself.

This is the phase of treatment in which your oncologist is going to be paying even more attention to symptoms and side effects of the cancer itself, even though you may be switching to a new line of therapy. If you have been on hormonal therapy, this might mean another hormonal agent, but this also might mean switching to chemotherapy. Switching to a different type of treatment can be an enormous adjustment. You may need to get to know a chemotherapy nurse and the rhythms of a chemotherapy infusion unit, for example.

One recent patient I worked with had a particularly difficult time with this. Gwen was a teacher in her late fifties with metastatic breast cancer and she had responded extremely well to several years of hormonal therapy followed by more than a year of feeling well on chemotherapy. When she noticed that she was having a new pain in her right side, scans showed that the cancer was getting worse. Gwen was switched to a new chemotherapy, but within four months the cancer was clearly getting worse. I explained that she was in a different phase of treatment, in which the cancer would be harder to control, and Gwen told me that she understood. The next week, she came into the clinic complaining of abdominal discomfort. I told Gwen that I wanted to start her on some pain medication, and she seemed shocked. She told me that she fully expected that the tumors would shrink again once she had started the new regimen because that is what had happened for years on treatment. Of course, I hoped that this would be true and that she would have a good response to this next line of treatment. But, as her oncologist, I also worried about what would happen if the treatment didn't work as well as we both hoped. I wanted her to understand that we had to stay on top of new symptoms so that she wouldn't struggle with them over time. In retrospect, I realized that this was the first time Gwen really began to understand that her cancer was incurable.

A second line of treatment is usually second because research shows that it is less likely than the first line to control the cancer in most patients. The same is true for a third line. It's at this point in treatment that your oncologist may be starting to get worried about the ability of the chemotherapy or hormonal therapy to control your cancer. Every cancer is a bit different, and some people, especially those with a hormone receptor–positive or HER2-postive tumor, can get a good response from several lines of therapy. However, sometimes the cancer doesn't respond the way we are hoping it will.

At this point in time it is important to remember that you didn't fail the therapy. People like to think that they somehow control the good responses, through diet or exercise or supplements or meditation. If they believe that logic, then when a line of treatment doesn't work, they believe that they didn't do something correctly. Cancer is biological just like an infection. If you had a urinary tract infection, and it stopped responding to a particular antibiotic, you would try a new antibiotic. We do the same thing in cancer treatment. If the one drug doesn't work as well as another, there is a biological explanation. Your tumor is resistant to the biological pathway that a particular therapy uses to attack the cancer cells.

Resistance to Targeted Therapy

Some patients have been taking targeted therapies for months or years with extraordinary results before the cancer becomes resistant. Vicki worked with a patient, Patsy, who had HER2-positive breast cancer. The HER2 gene was one of the first targets that was discovered in cancers and it was a major breakthrough when it was discovered that antibodies directed at the HER2 protein could cause the cancers to shrink dramatically. Patsy had been on trastuzumab for over three years and her cancer that had been widespread when she first responded melted like butter. She felt terrific for three years, and then one day came in with headaches and a drooping eyelid. An MRI of her brain revealed that little clumps of tumor had begun to grow on the lining covering her brain. It turns out that many women with HER-amplified breast cancers will experience brain metastases. Trastuzumab doesn't get into the brain very well and doctors often refer to the brain as a "sanctuary site" where breast cancer cells can hide for years. Patsy had some radiation and started chemotherapy, but it wasn't as effective. It was a heartbreaking transition for Patsy to go from feeling nearly normal to having brain metastases that were hard to treat. She told Vicki that it was like being diagnosed all over again.

Best- and Worst-Case Scenarios

This is a good time to ask your oncologist to give you an idea about the best- and worst-case scenarios for this new line of treatment. The situation changed because the cancer has become resistant to one or more drugs, and you will want to get a picture of what the future might hold at this time. There is still a lot of uncertainty, but this might be a time when the best-case scenario is measured in months rather than years.

Sometimes when a patient changes to a new line of therapy, she may feel sicker from the cancer or because the body has already endured many prior treatments and interventions. This can be a tough time for some patients because they feel their body isn't tolerating the infusions or the medications in the same way. Other patients do well even though their cancer is still slowly growing through treatment. It is different for everyone. Your oncologist can't predict how you will respond to this new line.

Whenever you switch to a new line of therapy, your doctor will review with you the likely side effects of the new drugs. They should also let you know that more cancer treatment isn't always better and that there may come a time when the treatment can shorten your life rather than extend it.

Symptom Management

At this time, your medical team members should be asking you a lot of questions about how you feel physically. They will be paying particular attention to your blood counts and to pain and fatigue, and they will review with you the signs of infection and the signs of any bleeding issues. This is the time to pick up the phone and call the clinic or your doctor if anything seems off or if you are struggling to manage your symptoms at home. Your oncologist and nurse practitioner want to work actively with you to adjust any medications and keep you feeling your best. I always ask people how they are sleeping, what they do during the day, and how their bodies respond to the infusions. As cancer progresses, we pay particular attention to pain management, neurologic issues, difficulties with breathing, and fatigue.

Pain Management

Some patients notice a change in the intensity of pain as their cancer progresses. Cancer can spread to the bones, or it can spread to abdominal organs and tissues, which might make it more difficult to move or sleep comfortably. Even if you have avoided pain medication to this point, your doctor might encourage you to manage your pain actively. If you have been taking pain medication, your doctor will be asking whether it's still working. We worry at this time about opioid tolerance and about intractable pain, which means pain that's not responding to opioids.

Tolerance to Opioids

Patients who have taken opioids for pain for some time may have noticed that the doses have increased over time. That's normal and expected as long as the pain can be managed by higher doses. If at some point you are taking long-acting opioids and still need several doses of short-acting pain medication to handle breakthrough pain, your doctor may wonder whether you have developed some tolerance for the opioids you are taking. This means that your brain has increased the number of receptors for that specific kind of opioid. Patients sometimes experience this if they have slow-growing tumors and have been in treatment for several years. The usual fix is to increase the dose or try a different pain medication. Doctors call the process of switching drugs an *opioid rotation*.

One patient at the clinic, Jill, had a slow-growing breast cancer that had spread to her bones. She was doing great with hormonal therapy. Her tumor markers (levels of proteins secreted by cancer cells; see chapter 6) remained low, and her CT scans showed stable disease. Despite the stability of the cancer, her bone pain increased over a period of two months. With her oncologist's guidance, she tried increasing her short-acting oxycodone for immediate pain relief. Then they increased her Oxycontin, her long-acting medication. The pain would respond for a couple of days to these newer doses and then return. Her doctor then switched her to a different medication, in this case a fentanyl patch, to help with ongoing pain, and gave her hydromorphone for those times when the pain increased sharply. Within one week, she was feeling much more comfortable.

When you change your opioid medication, you will have to work closely with your oncologist or palliative care specialist. There will be some experimentation to find the right dose of the new medication. Sometimes I ask patients to be admitted to the hospital to do this because we can give IV medications while the nurses are supervising you. We can find the appropriate dose much more quickly that way.

Treatments for Intractable Pain

In those cases where pain management becomes an ongoing issue, we sometimes think of using intravenous medications instead of oral opioids or pain patches. This doesn't mean staying in the hospital hooked up to an IV. Patients can use something called *patient-controlled analgesia*, which is a pump often used by people recovering from surgery. It comes with a button you can push to deliver more pain medication as needed. This is a wonderful tool that gives people a sense of control over their own medication while living at home.

Another option is something called intrathecal pain medication, which is sort of like having an epidural during childbirth. The pain specialist will insert a tiny catheter into the spine in an area that will give the patient the most relief. Then he or she will fill a pump that is also implanted inside the body. The benefit is that the pump sends pain medication, such as an opioid, directly to the affected nerves and keeps them from sending pain signals to the brain. As a result, you can reduce the level of opioid pain medication and the side effects that come with them. The downside is that it's cumbersome to use. A pain specialist has to refill the pump, and, because it's inside your body, it can become a source for infection. Doctors tend to recommend this option when escalating doses of oral or IV medications don't provide relief or come with intolerable side effects.

Always remember that radiation to a particular location of cancer can result in dramatic improvements in pain control. This is particularly useful for cancers that are in the bone or cancers that are pressing against a nerve.

Fatigue

Most people experience increased fatigue after their cancer stops responding to treatment. Early on in treatment, you may have experienced fatigue from the chemotherapy or radiation treatments but bounced back after a few days. As the cancer spreads, you may have to ration your energy more carefully.

Allie was a nurse who had metastatic breast cancer and initially did remarkably well with chemotherapy. She had no pain, no nausea, and no shortness of breath. Initially she was able to keep her job in a pediatric clinic. As her cancer progressed, she struggled with fatigue and had trouble putting in a full day at work. Allie told me that she had prepared to suffer from her cancer with pain or nausea but that she never quite realized the suffering that would come from fatigue. It physically pained her that she was too tired to keep working or even interact with people on a regular basis. Unfortunately, fatigue caused by cancer is very hard to control. If you can't control it, you have to work around it. Vicki often tells people to take note of those times of day when they feel most energetic and plan to do important tasks during those times. Save your energy for those things that matter most.

Other Treatment Options

Advancing cancer is a time when patients and families ask about alternative therapies. Some take a new interest in nutritional supplements, which Vicki discussed in chapter 13, and others wonder about experimental drugs in other countries and ask whether there isn't something else to try. Or they ask about expensive overseas clinics that mix alternative therapies with standard care. (In chapter 22, we explain why doctors advise against this.)

New experimental drugs are being tested all the time, and the best way to get access to them is to enroll in a clinical trial. But a clinical trial isn't for everyone. For some, it means traveling to a clinical research center, which may be expensive or inconvenient. Others simply have an immediate aversion to the idea. They don't want to take drugs that are still being tested. They don't want to be a test pilot flying a new kind of airplane. They want only standard, proven treatments, and that's great. A clinical trial is just an option, though sometimes participating in one is the only way to access new treatments for your disease.

Clinical Trials

Before you decide if a clinical trial is the right option for you, you should know how they work and what each phase of a trial hopes to accomplish.

Phase I. This is sometimes called a first-in-human study. Researchers who have tested a promising new treatment in the lab need to find out whether it is tolerable in humans and at what dose it might be effective. Phase I trials typically enroll patients with advanced cancers for whom the standard treatments are no longer working. Because we have no idea if this drug will help a particular patient, we often think about participation in these as a generous and important gift to science and the care of others living with breast cancer.

Phase II. These typically enroll between 30 and 50 patients who will receive the same dose and schedule of a new drug that has completed phase I testing. In this phase, doctors are still testing the safety of a new drug, but they will also measure how effectively it either shrinks the cancer or keeps it stable. We call this the response rate. It's always good to ask the physicians running the trial what they would consider a success in this clinical trial. This will give you a good idea of what to expect.

Phase III. These are randomized trials, meaning that you will be randomly enrolled in one of two arms, or groups of patients, of the study. A computer assigns you to receive either standard care alone or standard care plus the new drug. You don't get to choose which arm of the study you will join, but you may know whether you are receiving the new treatment or not, and so will your doctors. At this point, researchers are comparing the efficacy of the new treatment to standard care. Some studies contain a placebo arm, meaning neither the patient nor the doctor knows whether you are taking the new drug or getting standard care.

You don't need to be frightened by clinical trials. Instead, you can ask your oncologist which studies are going on for patients with your type of breast cancer. This should prompt a good discussion about the current standard of care and what kind of drugs are emerging for your type of cancer. It is important to know that participation in some clinical trials may mean more visits to the hospital and additional testing. Ask your team about what each trial entails to see if it seems like a good fit for you.

While enrolling in a clinical trial can be an appropriate option at any point, it tends to be more of an option as cancer worsens. You don't have to be treated at a teaching hospital to participate in one of these studies, either. Clinical research takes place in many nonacademic settings.

Informed Consent

Many people agonize over the decision to enroll in a clinical trial or study. Before you consent, your oncologist will explain what the study is and describe what's known about the new drug. They will tell you about the possibility of toxicity and also describe exactly what the study will measure. In some cases, researchers are hoping to extend life expectancy for just a few extra months, or they are hoping for a response rate that is slightly higher than that of standard care. For some people, this is a difficult conversation because it highlights the fact that their cancer has progressed to the point where standard care can't control it anymore and that even the newest treatments won't bring a cure.

Dave remembers conducting one of these conversations early in his career. Hazel was a 68-year-old woman with metastatic breast cancer who was trying to decide whether to enroll in a clinical trial for a new chemotherapy drug. Her cancer had grown through the first line of treatment, and she seemed very interested in the idea of receiving a new drug. Dave explained to her in technical terms what they were hoping to measure in the study: a response rate that was 30% instead of 20% and to extend progression-free survival by two to three months. Hazel smiled at Dave and said that she was hoping for a cure. Dave smiled back at her and explained again what the study would measure. They had this exchange a couple of times before Hazel stopped and said, "You think I didn't hear you the first time?" She said, "I'm allowed to hope and you're not allowed to take that away from me." She was right. Dave says he thought she wasn't listening to him. Instead, Dave realized that he was the one not listening to her.

In this discussion, you can and should ask a lot of questions about the study, how it will be conducted, and what life might look like as a participant. If you do enroll, you should know that your life will be busier than it is in standard care. You will meet regularly with a clinical research nurse who is responsible for the conduct of the trial and who will make sure that the oncologist is doing everything exactly as the protocols dictate. You may have extra blood tests to document how quickly the drug clears out of your system (called pharmacokinetics) and extra scans and other tests to determine how the drug is affecting your body (called pharmacodynamics). Behind the scenes, a clinical research coordinator will collect all the data from your tests and scans and document in exhaustive detail your progress throughout the trial. They will also make sure that regulatory documents have been filled out.

Before you can enroll, too, the oncologist will have to get your informed consent. This entails a long discussion about every aspect of the trial and everything that will be expected of you, and you will need to sign a document stating that you understand everything about the study and the risks involved. You should have a good understanding of all of these facts before you sign a consent document. You should also understand that you can withdraw your consent at any time during the study without fear of any repercussions. This is one of the first principles of medical ethics when it comes to clinical trials.

Family Meetings

Some people try to hide the news that their cancer is progressing from family and close friends, telling themselves that they don't want to burden anyone. Countless patients have told us that they will tell their adult children about this later, at some future point, but that point never seems to come. And then we get phone calls from these close family members demanding to know what's going on. They are often in tears, and they feel hurt or betrayed by the patient's silence. By law, doctors cannot disclose information about a patient to anyone without the patient's permission. So, at this point, I often suggest a family meeting, which is a chance for the patient, the medical team members, and key family members to sit in the same room and discuss the treatment plan.

You can request a family meeting at any time, but these can be especially powerful when your treatment options are changing or when the cancer is beginning to grow through the treatments. Your doctor can help you break the news to family members and talk in concrete terms about next steps. Your doctor can lay out the best-case scenario and the worst-case scenario, just as he or she did when you were first diagnosed. For patients, this is a chance to say to everyone what you want and don't want in terms of treatment and for everyone to hear your wishes. It's easy to believe that information will worry people, but the truth is that your family already feels concerned about what is happening and about what might happen next, and silence only makes their anxiety worse.

CHAPTER TWENTY

Living and Hoping with Advancing Cancer

I (Vicki) often meet with patients for the first time in my capacity as a palliative care doctor after they have been told that their cancer is incurable or that it has begun to grow despite treatment. In either case, the news is shocking and often feels surreal. For those in active treatment, they have worked hard to become capable cancer patients. Most of them have figured out a system for dealing with the side effects of treatment and have continued to work or volunteer. They have lived as normally as possible for many months or several years. Perhaps they have gone on trips and spent extra time with their families. And they have focused on everything their oncologist has focused on, which is getting through treatments with the hope that the cancer will continue to be held in check.

It's disorienting to be told that treatments are no longer keeping the cancer from spreading, even when you have been through multiple lines of chemotherapy, even when you have had a health crisis that shows the spread of tumors (metastases) to new areas of the body, and even when you feel a lot of fatigue. It's difficult to understand what might happen next, no matter how much you know about your diagnosis.

For example, I worked closely with Michelle who was diagnosed with stage 3 breast cancer at the age of 52. She worked in a hospital as an administrator and was pretty savvy about medical care. She had a lumpectomy and radiation followed by chemotherapy. Afterward, she had no evidence of disease for three years. She knew that her diagnosis had been serious but was very hopeful that the aggressive treatment had meant that she was cured. After her cancer did recur, Michelle told her oncologist that she refused to think about the fact that she might die. She responded very well to chemotherapy for over two years. After her first line of chemo stopped working, and then the second line, she got frustrated with her oncologist. The truth was that she had trouble believing that the cancer was getting worse, even though she had multiple tumors in her liver and was struggling to manage her fatigue enough to go to work.

Michelle was a smart, dedicated professional, and yet she needed help understanding what was happening in her body. A lot of people do.

In this chapter, I describe some strategies you can use to cope with this confusion and the anxiety that comes with it. In palliative care we talk about a concept called prognostic awareness, and I explain what that is. But we also talk a lot about hope—and what to hope for in this challenging time. You can continue to hope and to make plans, even if you aren't hoping for a cure.

What Is Prognostic Awareness?

At many points after diagnosis, people wonder whether they might die from cancer. Early on in treatment, it's easier to push these thoughts away and pretend they don't exist. Sometimes they pop up again when you are awake at 3:00 a.m. or when you are alone and feeling down. Even when these thoughts become consuming, most people don't share them with anyone. It can feel disloyal to talk about the possibility of death with people who are working to support you while you are going through treatment.

During my first appointment with Michelle, we talked about a lot of subjects, including pain management, fatigue, and finding some ways for her to continue to work, which she really loved. Then I asked her what she hoped for and what she was worried about. For some people, this is the first time anyone has asked this question and actually wanted to hear the answer.

"I'm terrified that I might die from this," she said. Michelle believed that optimism was the only thing that was keeping her cancer in check. She was afraid that she would be letting her family and friends down if she admitted that she had moments of real sadness. Although she told her family and her doctor that she was going to beat this, she actually worried constantly about the cancer getting worse.

In fact, Michelle was afraid that saying anything out loud about dying was inviting her cancer to get worse. But there is no data to suggest that this is true. Talking about it doesn't make it happen. In fact, all the energy you exert trying not to think about or talk about it can be exhausting. You should not be sitting with these worries all alone.

The process of understanding your illness is called prognostic awareness, and it takes time to develop. You don't have to make sense of all of this difficult information about the future all at once. You can and should do it in stages. The first stage is having a conversation about what you hope for and what you worry about. Over many subsequent conversations with Michelle, I asked her to think about and talk about what might happen. What if the disease got worse? What would that mean, and what decisions would we need to think about together? What if she had to stop working? What if she was hospitalized? Talking about these issues doesn't mean they are going to happen. But it's vital to have some safe place to think out loud and to create a possible plan B. Your care team can help you start these conversations.

There is a lot of uncertainty with serious cancer. Circumstances can change slowly over time, or they might change quickly. Most people need at least some sense of the future to inform their decisions about future treatments. That's why having some prognostic awareness, some ability to talk about the future, is so critical.

Am I in Denial?

I also remind patients that they don't have to have prognostic awareness all the time. In palliative care, we think of this awareness as a pendulum that swings back and forth. One minute you think you've got a handle on it, and then the next minute you feel certain that the diagnosis is a big mistake and that the doctors are just wrong.

Patients sometimes ask me, "Am I in denial? Sometimes I just pretend that things are fine. I know that what we talk about is true, but I just don't want to think about it all the time." This is perfectly normal. It is impossible to live with a constant awareness that time is shorter than you had hoped. Few patients are completely in denial. And no matter how much prognostic awareness you have, there's still room to hope for a miracle.

I recently interviewed a doctor at Mass General, a patient of Dave's, who had progressive pancreatic cancer and was about to go home to hospice care. I wanted to videotape our conversation so that a group of medical trainees could learn more about what it's like to live with a serious illness. I knew Doug would be the perfect person to talk to young doctors about how it feels to go through this. I asked Doug what he expected for the future. He said, "I know we have to wait and see. I know it might be months. It might be weeks. I'm going to go home with hospice, but I sort of want to believe that there's a five percent chance that Dave is going to walk in here and say he's found the perfect thing for me."

Doug didn't feel this way because he lacked awareness about his illness. He was a doctor. He knew the facts and he was able to integrate what he was told. He felt it because he is human. The truth is that Dave and I wished the same thing, too. It is normal to understand and then forget. Making sense of all of this all at once is impossible.

Later on, Doug said something in the interview that will stay with me forever. He was addressing the young medical students that he knew would watch the video. "I have no regrets," he said. "Listen guys, we all get to go to the party. And it's our job to make that party as good as we can make it. We don't all get to leave the party at the same time. Some of us have to leave the party early. But that doesn't mean it wasn't a damn good party."

Am I Giving Up Hope?

Some people are reluctant to talk at all about the possibility of death. Families sometimes worry that having these conversations might make the patient depressed or give up on treatment. Patients also worry that once they acknowledge the possibility of dying then they will have to experience all of the feelings that come with that possibility all at once. Or they worry that they will have to immediately solve all of the logistical concerns and family concerns that come with that possibility. And so people tell themselves that talking about death in any context is the same thing as giving up hope.

Becoming more comfortable with the idea that this cancer may take your life someday is not giving up hope. On the contrary, denying a difficult truth can be exhausting and stressful. I helped to conduct an early intervention palliative care study to see how patients reacted when asked to talk about these issues in a manner that was not overwhelming. The study showed that the people who had a place to voice their concerns slowly over time had a better quality of life, a 50% lower rate of depression, and an increased chance of living longer than those who were not receiving early palliative care.

Won't My Oncologist Bring It Up?

Some clinicians are reluctant to bring up the subject of death with patients. And research shows that doctors and their patients sometimes collude to avoid these conversations. Remember that your clinical team is made up of professionals who also get attached to their patients. The doctors and nurses in oncology work so closely with patients and their families. The oncologists I've worked with truly love their patients and fervently hope that treatments will work. Giving the news that treatment isn't working anymore is really hard for them, too. While many of them are comfortable initiating conversations about the next phase of the illness, a few of them wait for patients to initiate conversations about death.

If you want more information about the likely future with your illness, raise these questions with your care team. You can ask many of the same questions I asked Michelle. What might happen next? What if the cancer gets worse? What would that be like? How long do people with my type of cancer usually live after the treatment stops working?

How Much Do I Want to Know?

I always ask people to think about what kind of information would be helpful to know and when. There are no right or wrong answers. I've found that people think very differently about medical treatments if they have years to live rather than months or weeks. With more knowledge, they can make practical plans, such as whether to take a vacation or change the date of a family event to make more certain that they can attend. Or they want to know specifically whether they are likely to be alive for a major holiday or life event, such as a child's or grandchild's graduation.

Other people are less interested in how much time they might have and instead want to know more about how they might feel as the illness progresses. Will I have more fatigue? Will I be able to work much longer? How much support will I need at home?

How Much Time Do I Have?

If you do ask your doctor to tell you how long you might live, be aware that no doctor can be completely certain about this. Typically, doctors think in terms of a range of possible outcomes, perhaps measured in years, months, or weeks. Another way that clinicians talk about the future is in terms of best-case, worst-case, and most likely scenarios. Sometimes the best-case scenario is also the most likely, but sometimes it isn't.

I like to tell patients what I am hoping for and what I am worried about. A patient of mine, Liz, was about to go home to hospice care. She was quite ill from her cancer. Liz asked me how long I thought she had. She had two teenagers, one of whom was going to graduate from high school in two months. At the time, I was worried it could be as short as a few weeks. I told her I hoped that I was wrong and that it was more like months. As it turns out, she had a delayed response to chemotherapy and the tumors stopped growing. We disenrolled her from hospice so that she could start a new treatment regimen, and she lived another nine months. When she came back to see me at the clinic for help with her pain management, I asked her how she felt about my inaccurate estimate. Liz smiled at me. "You said you hoped you would be wrong and you were. I figured you were just really happy that you were wrong. I got to prepare everyone in case I couldn't be there for Kara's graduation," she said. It's true. I was so happy to be wrong, and Liz wasn't disappointed in me because I was wrong. She found that having the information that her time might be quite short helped her to prepare her family.

It is the fear of being inaccurate that keeps so many clinicians from these discussions about time. I find that most people just want to know in broad terms what their doctor thinks is likely. They don't hold us to it, but it gives them a range that is helpful.

Sometimes you ask for information about how long you might live and then struggle to remember what was said. It can be difficult to process this information the first time you hear it. I had a patient named Tammy who had lived for years with breast cancer that was only in her bones. She had really become accustomed to living life with breast cancer. It didn't cause her too much trouble and she could put it out of her mind most of the time. Unfortunately, Tammy started developing headaches and noticed that her left-hand grip felt weaker and that she had trouble picking up a mug of coffee. She was then diagnosed with leptomeningeal disease, which is when the cancer spreads to the lining around the brain. It is very hard to treat and can become serious quite fast. Tammy and I met with her oncologist, and at this meeting Tammy asked whether she would be alive for Christmas, which was three months away. Her oncologist said that Christmas was a stretch, but that she had a good shot of making it to her birthday, which was in one month.

Later that day, Tammy told her oncology nurse that the senior oncologist had told her that she had between six and eight months to live. Then when Tammy's daughter came to see her, Tammy told her that she didn't know what the future would hold and that she just wanted to take things in two-week increments. Was Tammy in denial all day? Probably not. She was slowly acclimating to a very difficult reality. Integrating information like this takes time, and not everyone can hear a piece of information like this and hang onto it.

Can I Change My Mind?

It's also perfectly okay to change your mind and to want more information at one point and less later on. I worked with a patient named Diane who was in her seventies and living with triple-negative breast cancer whose future with the illness was uncertain. She would sometimes ask me a question about the future and then stop herself, saying, "On second thought. I don't want to know." She told me that the cancer is what it is and that she and her family would have to figure things out as they happened. I knew that Diane had good prognostic awareness. She wasn't refusing to talk about the future because she thought the doctors were wrong or because she thought that she would still be cured. Instead, she knew that having a lot of information about different potential developments wouldn't be helpful for her in her goal of living her life fully. She wanted to focus on the activities that she could still do that she still loved to do.

About a year later, Diane was hospitalized with liver failure due to tumors in her liver, and she asked me to tell her exactly how long I thought she had to live and what that time might be like. I asked her why she wanted this information because she had been so adamant about not talking about it before. Diane told me that she worried that her children didn't understand how sick she was. "I feel that I need to know more now so that I can tell them," she said. So we had a long conversation about the likely trajectory of her illness, and she shared that information with her children. She wanted to know whether she had weeks or months to live so that she could make plans and help her children prepare.

In our most recent visits, Diane has told me that she wants to go back to not talking about the future. She has even told her oncologist that she doesn't want to know the results of her CT scans. "We are where we are," she said to me. "What good does it do me?"

There are times when the person living with cancer wants more or less information than the family wants, too. You can probably work out a plan where the doctor will have a slightly different conversation with you than he or she has when family are present. Sometimes people living with cancer want to take things as they come, while family members want more detailed information about what might happen next so they can plan for hospice care or family leave. Sometimes the patient really wants to know all the available information about the future, but the family doesn't. I usually ask both the patient and the loved ones what information would be helpful and defer to the patient's preferences. Sometimes the patient asks that I talk with the family, but they don't want to know. That is fine with me as long as the patient is okay with it.

Coping without Getting Down

As my patients begin to hold a deeper understanding of the likely illness trajectory, it can be hard to know how to cope effectively and stay focused on living fully. It doesn't help when other people spout annoying platitudes because they don't know what else to say. Some people tell my patients simplistic things, such as, "Live each day to the fullest!" One of my patients had this sarcastic reply: "Sure. I'll get right on that." Another patient said, "Seriously? Why don't you try it sometime?"

The truth is that people with advancing cancer are living with a foot in two worlds. They live in the world with their family and friends where they want to make plans and accomplish goals. But they also live in a world where they have a sense that life is going to be different from what they'd hoped for. This is a sad, often painful, reality.

I remind people at this time that feeling down is normal. One of my patients insisted to me that she was depressed and told me that she was sobbing the day before because she could no longer take her long daily walks. Her neuropathy had become so bad that she could no longer play her favorite pieces on the piano. The cancer was taking things away from her that she really loved to do. When I asked her how she spent her time, she told me that she visits her grandchildren every chance she gets. They watch silly movies together and play games. She spends time with her friends. I had to tell her that just because you are sad doesn't mean you are depressed. She was clearly able to find joy in life, and it was okay for her to feel sad about what she could no longer do.

My patients tell me that it is most helpful if they give themselves and their family members permission to just forget about the illness at times. When they do talk to loved ones about difficult subjects, they give cues for when they are ready to talk about something serious, and they limit those conversations. When they've had enough, they say so. And that gives everyone the signal that it's time to talk about other matters and maybe forget about the illness if they can.

People who cope especially well at this time are the people who keep making plans that help them look forward to something in the future. I always ask people what they are looking forward to. It might be a visit to see family or a walk on the beach. It could be anything—a tour of major ballparks, a woodworking project, or a hobby you have hoped to engage in more fully. Now is the time. It is critical to keep a forward momentum.

Having a practice of gratitude can also be helpful. Even in the midst of something as difficult as cancer, people can develop an appreciation for this new perspective on life. Some people start to think in terms of gratitude for those they love and their work and their spiritual community. Instead of thinking solely about all that they have lost to the cancer, they try to notice everything they have, including the support of good friends, work they love, their spiritual life, or even a devoted pet. My patients tell me that focusing on what they have and what they love is a powerful antidote for the feeling that cancer is running their lives.

Some of my patients do something that I still find amazing. They express gratitude for aspects of their illness. One patient, Joe, recently said to me, "I would never have asked for this. Never. But I can't deny that everything is different for me. I love my wife more. I could just sit and watch my kids play for hours. This spring when the blossoms came out on the trees, I saw how magnificent they were. I'd never appreciated that before. I know it sounds corny, but I don't take things for granted the way I used to."

Joe is unusual. Having cancer doesn't automatically make you appreciate everything more, and you don't have to try to do that if it's not your style. People like Joe understand the burdens of cancer. They know how much treatment has encroached on their autonomy. But they can still stay curious about how this new perspective has changed their relationships, and through this curiosity they are better able to partner with the cancer. They don't have to think of it solely as an enemy, and they don't have to think in terms of winning or losing a battle. They look for ways to say, "I'm still me. This is still my life."

CHAPTER TWENTY-ONE

What about Practical Concerns?

Some people will have an oncologist say to them that they need to get their affairs in order. It can be hard to figure out exactly what that means beyond meeting with an accountant, if appropriate, or having a current will. You may want to create a spreadsheet with account numbers for insurance policies and passwords for email accounts and bank accounts, and you may want to communicate your wishes for any funeral arrangements. These discussions with family members can be fraught with anxiety because the people who love and support you may say they prefer to not talk about these things. But we have found that these same family members will have an easier time later on if you've been firm with them about making arrangements while you still feel well enough to organize these details.

Think of this chapter as a way of taking some unpleasant medicine that will make things better, even though you may have to figure out how to get it down. When you have a serious illness like cancer, there is some really basic planning that you can get out of the way, knowing you will feel better about it afterward.

Choosing a Health Care Proxy

Assign someone to make medical decisions for you if necessary. This may be called a health care proxy or a durable power of attorney for health care. It's a legal document that you must sign, and in some states you need an attorney to draw up the forms. In other states, you can download a form and fill it out as long as witnesses sign with you.

When you chose someone to act as a health care proxy, make sure this person knows you well and will be able to make decisions as you would. You want to choose someone who lives near you and can travel easily to a hospital to make these decisions and someone who will be a strong advocate for your wishes even in the presence of conflicting opinions from family members or friends.

Have a detailed conversation with this person about whether you would want to be maintained on a breathing machine and under what circumstances you wouldn't want your life prolonged. Talk about what quality of life means to you, and identify the kind of life you would want to avoid. You have to be clear about your goals and values. What in your life is so important to you that you can't imagine living without it? Do you want life prolonged if you have untreatable pain? What do we do if you suddenly got sick and were on a breathing machine but we didn't think you could get better?

For some people, a spouse is the likely choice for the role of health care proxy. In fact, if you signed a living will years ago, you may have already assigned this role to your spouse. You may need to review your will and make sure that this decision still makes sense. A spouse may not be the right choice if he or she cannot make objective decisions for you.

Life-Sustaining Treatment Forms

Many patients hire an attorney to create a living will that outlines their goals and values and may even state specific wishes about medical treatment at the end of life. While it's a great idea to do this, you should remember that a living will does not translate into a medical order for treatment. In most states you need to fill out an additional form and have a doctor sign it. This form might be called Medical Orders for Life-Sustaining Treatment (MOLST) or Physician Orders for Life-Sustaining Treatment (POLST). This form dictates how much treatment you should get in a life-threatening emergency, and that one form is valid no matter where you are—in a hospital or in a rehab facility or at home.

Without one of these forms, you will be considered "full code," meaning that medical professionals must do everything possible to keep you alive, even if you are not conscious and are not likely to regain consciousness. In Massachusetts, the forms are usually bright pink to make them easy for paramedics to find. Once you have filled out a POLST or MOLST form, you should make sure the people who are caring for you can retrieve it easily. Most people don't know that an emergency medical technician (EMT) or emergency room nurse will assume that every patient is full code and attempt resuscitation unless someone can produce these medical orders. People generally keep these forms along with the health care proxy and durable power of attorney forms in an envelope affixed to the refrigerator and marked as "medical forms." EMTs know to look on the fridge for these forms.

You will want to have a conversation with your oncologist before filling out one of these forms as well. You can ask directly whether cardiopulmonary resuscitation (CPR) or intubation will help you as your cancer progresses. Resuscitation is a medical procedure in which the patient receives interventions in the hope of restarting the flow of blood and oxygen throughout the body. It involves medication, chest compressions, electric shocks to the chest, and the insertion of a breathing tube. Unfortunately, we know from studies that these medical interventions don't work well in patients who have progressive, metastatic cancer.

It's unsettling to have to talk about death and to sign a form issuing medical orders. We always remind patients that signing one of these orders doesn't mean doctors won't do anything for you. Your medical team will still be working to improve your health, to make sure you are as comfortable as possible and free of distress. They can still give you radiation for pain, drain fluid from your lungs, if needed, and give you supplemental oxygen.

Some patients tell us they want their doctors to make the decisions about whether to attempt CPR or insert a breathing tube if there is a medical crisis. Unfortunately, it doesn't work that way. Medical professionals must take life-sustaining measures unless you have filled out the life-sustaining treatment form to indicate otherwise, even if your quality of life isn't what you want, even if the interventions cause you pain or distress. We caution patients that when you have progressive, metastatic cancer, resuscitation probably won't be effective. CPR and intubation won't affect the underlying cancer that has triggered the medical crisis.

Occasionally, a patient will say they want the doctors to try ventilation for a while and then remove the machines after a few days if things don't get better. It sounds reasonable, and yet most oncologists and palliative care specialists don't usually recommend short-term ventilation. When you make decisions, you also want to think of your family members and what they will be feeling in this situation. Once you are on a ventilator, someone has to decide to remove the machines, and that's a gut-wrenching decision for someone to have to make on your behalf. A growing body of research suggests that when someone's death is prolonged in the intensive care unit, their family members struggle more with grief and post-traumatic stress.

We suggest patients ask their doctors several questions: "Will the resuscitation allow me to live the quality of life that is acceptable to me?" and "Given what you know about me and about my cancer, what would you recommend?" A doctor should give you a recommendation about these kinds of medical interventions just as they would recommend medications for you to take.

End-of-Life Care

We often encourage patients to start thinking about what they want at the end of life and about the circumstances in which they wouldn't want life prolonged. There is a growing awareness in our culture that everyone should think and talk about end-of-life care, what each one of us would want and not want if we had a medical crisis that diminished our quality of life as we see it. But these conversations have even more relevance for patients with advancing cancer.

The Conversation Project is a nonprofit started by journalist Ellen Goodman to help initiate these discussions. The goal of the project is to help people talk about their wishes for end-of-life care. Goodman started the project after providing end-of-life care for her mother and realizing that very few people talk to their close family members about what kind of care they would want if their health deteriorated. It starts with asking what your priorities are. Making a statement to your family about what matters to you, what brings you joy in life, is the first step. There are many other questions to answer about how much detail you want about your medical condition and whether you are more afraid of having too much care or too little. You can visit websites together looking for information about how to determine your goals and values.

We initiate a lot of these conversations with our patients, and they always help people with cancer to think about what they want and don't want as treatments become more intensive. They think about quality of life and what matters so much to them that they couldn't imagine living without it. There aren't right or wrong answers. Everyone has a different answer to these questions.

One patient, named Theresa, was very clear with her family that living well with cancer meant being able to be engaged with her grandchildren and being active. If she needed to spend the whole day in bed, she didn't want that type of life prolonged. She was clear that she didn't want any more treatments that could cause fatigue, nausea, and pain. She didn't want treatments that would make her too sick to function. She was also clear that she wanted to die at home, and she didn't want any artificial measures to prolong her life. She was able to state what she really wanted and work with her family to make sure those wishes were carried out.

By contrast, another patient, named Alexandra, who also had three young children, stated clearly that she wanted every possible medical treatment for her breast cancer, even if that meant suffering on her part. We talked at length about her goals and values. She understood that she would most likely die from her cancer and knew that she didn't want to be resuscitated when she was close to death. Still, she wanted all experimental treatments attempted if they could be safely delivered. Alexandra started a clinical trial a month before her death, even though she had a do-not-resuscitate order in place. In the end, Alexandra believed that she had tried every possible medical treatment but also that she had made a plan for the end of her life that would support her and her family.

Choosing Hospice Care

Many people say they hope to die at home if possible, but not everyone wants this. Most patients say they want to be physically comfortable and don't want to be a burden to their family members. These patients consider the location of death secondary to these other concerns. We think it's great to know what you hope to do, and it's also good to stay flexible if you can't remain at home.

Your care team will encourage you to choose a home hospice provider to give you and your family more support. Hospice gets a bad reputation because so many patients think you can engage hospice only during the final days of life. As a result, they wait too long to get the help that would really be useful. Also some people think you have to stop all treatments and stop seeing your regular doctors when you enroll in hospice. This is not true. You may choose to see your doctors even when you are enrolled in hospice, as long as you are feeling strong enough to come to the clinic or to join a virtual visit.

Once you enroll in hospice, that hospice provider pays for all of your medical treatment. This includes medications, nursing and home health aide visits, and any medical equipment, such as hospital beds or oxygen. Hospice providers vary in which other services they are able to offer, however. Many smaller hospices can't cover such treatments as chemotherapy, which can cost upwards of $10,000 per month. Larger hospices tend to cover more treatments, and some are considered "open access" providers, meaning that patients can still receive such therapies as chemotherapy and radiation. There is one hospice provider in Massachusetts, in fact, that had more than 100 patients receiving chemotherapy at one point. Before enrolling, do some research to find a provider that can meet your needs. Look for a provider with physicians who are board-certified in hospice and palliative medicine.

When to Enroll in Hospice

We often have to explain to patients and families that hospice care is not just for people who are critically ill or actively dying. It's an insurance benefit available to patients with a likely prognosis of six months or less. (And if you live longer than six months, they don't kick you out.) The goal of hospice is to help you live well during these months.

Some patients in hospice have a remarkable amount of energy when they enroll, like Kara, who had lived with breast cancer for nearly 20 years. The cancer was growing and she had had so very many treatments. She was tired and didn't feel that more treatment made sense for her. She was the kind of person who had been very physically active. Before her cancer diagnosis she ran marathons and even when she developed tumors in her brain that made her a bit wobbly on her feet, she got a bike with three wheels so she could safely exercise. Her hospice nurse worked with her on taking her medications and managing her energy so that she could get out of the house and spend time with her family.

It's good to think of hospice as a kind of extension of palliative care. Hospice workers want to know your goals and help you live your life. One day, Kara had so much energy that she went out for a long bike ride with her sister and forgot that her nurse was scheduled to visit her. The nurse was worried when Kara did not answer the door. After reaching her, Kara said, "I'm sorry, but I have to get out of the house on nice days. Maybe we can go for a walk together the next time we have a beautiful day like today?"

One reason to enroll in hospice before you think you have a critical need for it is to get to know the people who will be coming to your home. Hospice is a group of providers assigned to you, including doctors, nurses, home health aides, social workers, chaplains, and volunteers. They work best when they have time to learn your routine so later on they can provide help more efficiently. A hospice nurse can come to your home up to three times per week, more if necessary, and will spend about an hour each visit. The home health aides can visit you as many as five days a week for about two to three hours at each visit. So, even if you have hospice, you will still rely on family and friends for the majority of your day-to-day needs. Hospice is not 24-hour home care. If you want that kind of care, you have to pay for it out of pocket or consider an inpatient hospice facility.

Inpatient Hospice

Most hospice care happens at home, but you can also receive hospice care in a hospice residence, nursing home, or hospital. The care delivered in a hospice residence is similar to the intensity of care that you can receive at home except there are caregivers there all the time to help with bathing, meals, and medications.

Most insurance plans do not cover residential hospice care, so the patient generally has to pay a daily rate. It could be as much as $200 to $500 per day. If you have symptoms that require a lot of monitoring or IV medication, then you need to be in an inpatient hospice facility or in the hospital. Fortunately, these stays are often covered by insurance. Your medical team can help you figure out what kind of care you need.

Some patients tour hospice houses to get a sense of where they would feel most comfortable. If you are feeling up to it, this is a great way to help your family decide what kind of care would be best. Your family members may be insisting that you stay at home—and it's wonderful to have a supportive family—yet the plan to stay at home doesn't work out for every patient. Sometimes symptoms are too hard to manage for family members. At some point in the future, you may need one or two people with you 24 hours a day, and that can be tough for some families to manage. If patients develop delirium or confusion, caring for them at home can be even more difficult. We like to encourage people to choose a hospice residence or general inpatient hospice unit as a backup plan. You can stay at home knowing that there is another option available if your family members are stretched too thin.

Funerals and Obituaries

Many people say that funerals are for the living, but that doesn't mean you have to leave all the details to others. And even though some people don't want to think about a possible funeral, others have a lot of opinions on the subject. They know whether they want to be buried or cremated. And they have ideas about where they want their ashes to be scattered or where they would like to be buried. Most people choose a place that has special meaning to them.

If you want your ideas and opinions known, you can visit a funeral home to start the planning process. Most are very good at helping families manage all these details, including open versus closed casket, planning a wake or memorial service, and whether to involve clergy or not. Many patients go to the funeral home to pick out such key items as a casket or an urn and to get help planning the services. If you can pay for the funeral in advance, this will be a great help to family members as well.

Vicki had a patient with aggressive metastatic breast cancer who was in her early forties. She had lived with her cancer for almost eight years and really wanted to take charge of her own funeral. She also had a quirky sensibility that was reflected in her choices of music, food, and who would speak at the service. She was very close to her niece and encouraged her to perform a funny skit at the funeral. "I want my funeral to be funny and silly like we are as a family," she said. "I wrote my obituary, too, and told people that if they can't take a joke, they shouldn't come to the funeral."

Managing Relationships

In the initial chapters on coping at the start of this book, Vicki talked about how to communicate changes in your health status to extended family and friends. It's no different now. You can think of your sphere of relationships as orbits, with orbit A at the center. Your A orbit is made up of those few people who know your situation well and are the ones providing the most day-to-day support. They know the details of your situation almost as soon as you do. And they can help explain it to others as needed.

The question is how you interact with outer orbits, what we call the B or C orbits. These are people you may love a lot and feel close to, but there are only so many times you can tell your story before you start to bore yourself. And, depending on your work history or social history, these outer orbits can consist of a lot of people who check in every few weeks and do want some sort of response or keep asking whether they can help. Be direct about what would be helpful to you and to your family. Maybe you simply want good wishes or prayers. Maybe you need help coordinating transportation or some food. People love to be given specific tasks they can do to help. It allows them to feel involved even when you aren't feeling especially social.

Some of our patients assign someone in their A orbit to serve as an information czar to their outer orbits. This is someone who likes writing group emails and is comfortable receiving messages and phone calls from people if they have questions. We usually recommend that this be someone other than a spouse or child of the patient, if possible. Immediate family members need to focus on themselves and the patient, and it can be exhausting to have the same conversation over and over again. If you use a website to manage meal donations or rides, your information czar can be in charge of that as well.

Having Important Conversations

Patients sometimes ask whether or how best to communicate love and gratitude to those closest to them. When you have a sense that time might be short, what do you say to the people you love? And some people want to know whether they should be trying to heal troubled relationships if possible. While there are no right or wrong answers, many palliative care clinicians have written about the kinds of conversations that help people feel some closure about the different relationships in their lives, and this helps them feel less anxious about death.

Ira Byock is a palliative care physician who has written several books on this subject, and he believes that these are conversations that everyone should have in order to heal. He identifies five phrases that may be helpful for people to say to loved ones: I'm sorry, I forgive you, thank you, I love you, and good-bye. This can seem formulaic for some people, and this list isn't for everyone, but it does offer a useful guide for how to initiate the kinds of conversations people might be grateful to have.

Legacy Work

One last practical question that patients sometimes ask about is how to create something tangible for or express something enduring to family members. For example, one patient who loved doing woodwork decided he wanted to build a cabinet for his wife, as a gift of his creativity. Some people want to work on specific projects with children or grandchildren, such as creating photo albums, assembling a family cookbook, or building model cars. Others buy gifts and attach messages to be opened at a significant event, such as a wedding or birthday, or they make videos in which they share memories and messages to loved ones, or they write letters. This is wonderful, meaningful work, but it can also be emotionally difficult, particularly when an illness is advanced and you are struggling with physical symptoms and fatigue. We would never tell anyone that they ought to do this work. It's different for everyone.

People who are very comfortable sharing their thoughts and feelings and have achieved some acceptance that cancer may take their lives at some point may find this work easier. They know that they should do it a little bit at a time on those days when they feel especially strong. One patient decided to write letters to her children in college about six months after her diagnosis, for example. Jane had metastatic breast cancer, and she wanted to start these letters early because she understood how much uncertainty the future held for her, and she wanted to share her thoughts with them and tell them how proud she was of them.

Jane was lucky to have a cancer that responded for some amount of time to nearly every treatment she was given, so she was able to live for much longer than expected. Every six months, she would come into the clinic and say, "I wasn't sure I would live this long, but I did. Now I have to rewrite those letters because there is so much more to say." She had a real knack for mock exasperation but knew that having to rewrite the letters was a great problem to have.

When writing her letters, Jane focused on highlighting stories about her children and her life that she remembered fondly, and she wrote a lot about what she loved and admired about her children. Although she had ideas about how she wanted them to live, she didn't focus on her own hopes. Children really do want to be seen and loved for who they are. They can feel burdened by letters filled with expectations about what career path they should choose or what kind of person they should marry. Instead, Jane focused on what it was like to hold each one of them for the first time and what memories of them she cherished most.

CHAPTER TWENTY-TWO

My Doctor Says Cancer Treatment Is No Longer Effective

Throughout the book, we have described how breast cancer that isn't curable will eventually spread and grow even though you are getting treatment. The timing of this is variable and will depend on the biology of your cancer and how many treatments your doctor has tried. Some hormone receptor–positive tumors may be controlled with various hormonal therapies for several years before eventually becoming resistant to these treatments, whereas other cancers may be treated with chemotherapy from the start and progress after just a few months of treatment. Either way, at some point treatments become less effective or even ineffective at controlling tumor growth.

If your tumor has progressed soon after starting a treatment or has progressed quickly through a couple of therapies in a row, oncologists start to worry about whether the tumor will be sensitive to further treatment. Even if there are other available drugs, they may work by a mechanism that the tumor has already grown resistant to. Also, the longer you are in treatment, the more likely your body will become weakened from the effects of the cancer and from multiple treatment regimens.

At some point, your oncologist is likely to tell you that continuing with cancer therapy may, in fact, shorten your life. Or perhaps your doctor will tell you that it simply won't do any good. (This situation is far different from taking a break early on when the treatment is working well. We sometimes refer to those as chemo holidays.)

It's never easy to hear that you won't be getting treatment for your cancer any more, but it is possible for these therapies to hurt you more than help you. This doesn't mean that you are weak or haven't tried hard enough. It just means that we can't do something that would do more harm than good.

It can be difficult to imagine how cancer treatments could be harmful to you, especially if it has been successful at holding the cancer in check for a long time. Some people demand to continue regimens of chemotherapy or other treatments even when the doctor has explained that they have only a remote chance of lengthening their lives even by a few weeks and a much larger chance of making them sick. People who are dealing with advanced cancer that has caused bone marrow failure and poor kidney or liver function are at higher risk for serious complications from treatment, and this is something oncologists want to avoid.

Even if your oncologist is telling you that you need to stop cancer treatment now, that doesn't mean that you can't have it ever again or that some other disease-modifying treatment won't be helpful to you in the future. In this chapter, we answer some of the questions that people have at this juncture and give you some guidelines for choosing treatments that are in line with your goals and values.

Are You Giving Up On Me?

Many times this is the first question patients ask their doctors when they are told that there are no more effective cancer treatments. The answer is absolutely not. Your doctors are still your doctors, and they will still be working with you to manage your cancer, minimize its symptoms, and help you with optimizing your quality of life.

In some cases, it is even harder for family members to make sense of this new reality. Many oncologists have been confronted by angry family members who say, "I forbid you to tell Mom that there aren't any other treatments." Spouses, too, have yelled at us, telling us that we've given up on a patient. Your doctors feel awful when this happens. We are not giving up. We just believe we would be bad doctors if we didn't prepare our patients and their families for what to expect. We always hope we're wrong, but we couldn't live with ourselves if we didn't help people understand what could happen if we continue with cancer treatments.

How Do You Know Chemotherapy Won't Be Effective?

We have a concept in oncology called performance status (PS). It's a rough rule of thumb that measures how patients feel during treatment. Your doctor will be giving you a PS rating between 0 and 4 at every appointment. If you have no side effects from cancer at all, you have a PS of 0. That means that you wouldn't even know that you had cancer if you weren't in treatment. If you have a PS of 1, you have some symptoms of cancer, but you can still function with good energy, and your daily activities haven't diminished significantly. Once you reach a PS of 2, you may find that you need to rest off and on during the day but are not spending more than half the day resting and conserving energy. A patient who has a PS of 3 is spending more than half the day in bed or on the couch. Once a patient is spending almost the whole day in bed and really struggles to summon the energy to function, that is a PS of 4.

Performance status measures how your body is responding to cancer therapies and how well it is able to bounce back after a treatment such as chemotherapy. It also serves as a rough measure of tumor burden, meaning the amount of cancer in the body. When patients have a PS of 3 or 4, the tumor burden may be high or the body has been knocked down by chemotherapy. Multiple clinical studies have shown that continuing to give these patients chemotherapy carries enormous risk and that these patients are unlikely to benefit from the treatment. As a result, oncologists are taught from the beginning of training that it's wrong to give chemotherapy to a patient with a PS of 3 or 4 if that patient has a solid tumor like breast cancer.

Stopping treatment applies mostly to chemotherapy decisions because patients with a borderline PS might still be safely treated with other such cancer therapies as the hormonal and HER2-targeted therapies. Talk to your doctor about what treatment options might be safe and effective for you and whether your PS rating might play a role in these decisions.

What Are My Options?

Sometimes patients sense before their doctors do that they've reached this juncture in treatment. They tell us that their fatigue is getting worse again or that they are losing weight. These are the classic signs that cancer is on the move. Sharon was a patient who had been living with metastatic breast cancer for three years when she got to this point. Her cancer had spread to her lungs and her shortness of breath had become one of the most reliable indicators of how she was doing. Over the previous month, she struggled to make it up a flight of stairs without stopping to catch her breath. One day in the clinic she said she already knew that the scans were going to show that the cancer was getting worse. She wanted to know what her options were.

This is a good time to have a conversation about treatment options and to ask your oncologist to go over the best- and worst-case scenarios for you. Some people ask, "How long have I got?" But even now an oncologist can't give you a definitive time frame. Instead we often talk about ranges of time, for example, months to years, weeks to months, or days to weeks. Because Sharon's cancer had been growing steadily in the past few months despite being treated with two types of chemotherapies, I (Jenn) estimated that she would likely have several months, or maybe less if her cancer started to progress more rapidly and caused deterioration in the functioning of her lungs.

In terms of other treatments, Sharon could have tried another breast cancer regimen that, on average, only delayed the growth of cancer for a couple of months and more often delivered no benefit. She could also have chosen a clinical trial for a drug that worked on her type of cancer in mice, but only a few people had been treated with the drug so far.

Her other choice was to not do any additional chemotherapy or clinical trials. Doctors call this supportive care. Many patients worry that this means doctors do nothing, but that's not true. Supportive care means helping patients have a good day each day. That sometimes requires interventions to remove fluid, radiation for pain, or other advanced symptom management. We still have many options to help patients live as well as they can. Your doctor may suggest home hospice at this point, because this will offer your family more support at home and the ability to get medications delivered there.

The next time Sharon came in to look at CT scans, she brought her husband, Phil. She looked grim when she said she had drawn up a new will and talked to their children about which of her family heirlooms she wanted each of them to have. And I knew this discussion was actually for Phil. For the next hour, I summarized for Phil the options Sharon and I had previously discussed. It was a difficult appointment for him, and at first he was insisting that she start the clinical trial right away. Eventually, he agreed that they should go home and discuss it first.

We have to remember that there are important goals other than living longer. *How* do you want to live? That is the most critical question at this point.

What Is a Marginally Effective Drug?

When people have exhausted standard chemotherapy, it can be compelling to try some other drug. It can be hard to understand that cancer cells mutate in ways that make them resistant to whole classes of standard treatments. And that means that even promising new drugs may not be effective against cancer cells that have gone through these mutations.

Even if your doctor knows of another line of chemotherapy, they may warn you that it will have only a small chance of being effective in your case. Oncologists refer to these drugs as being only marginally effective, meaning that they probably have less than a 10% or 20% chance of shrinking the cancer or controlling it for several months. Cancers that have already grown through several standard treatments are less likely to respond to each additional therapy, and yet the new drug will still bring side effects that patients will have to deal with. I always ask patients whether they truly want to do that or whether they want to try a different approach of supportive care.

The thought of stopping treatment may seem unbearable at first, but many people know that they only want to try another regimen with another set of side effects if it's going to be effective in keeping the cancer under control for several months or longer.

What about Experimental Drugs?

Doctors hear this question a lot. When you ask about other drug treatments, your doctor may suggest clinical trials, even phase I trials, in which drugs are being tested on people for the first time. These drugs will have shown promise in animal models in the lab, and they may be available to you if you qualify for such a study. But the decision to take part in a phase I trial is personal, and you'll want to consider what your goals are beyond the notion of living longer. In many studies of experimental chemotherapy, the goal is to improve longevity, perhaps by a few weeks or months. The goal is not to cure the cancer but to test and measure better treatments that could help others in the future.

I had a patient named Yvonne who was a 78-year-old accountant with metastatic breast cancer. She had spent her whole life working for herself in a small business that she owned. When her tumor had grown through standard chemotherapy options, we had a long talk about whether she should join a phase I study of a novel drug that showed promise in the lab against her type of cancer. The preclinical evidence looked great, but this trial was the first time that people would be taking it. So far, just five people had tried the drug, and it was too early to see how effective it would be. What impressed me about Yvonne was that she could look beyond the notion of experimental treatment and think clearly about how she wanted to spend the time she had left. She told me that she had always wanted to live at her Cape Cod house and redesign the swimming pool with her daughter who was inheriting the home. She knew that she had four or five good hours each day in which she could focus on a task. Yvonne told me that if she spent those hours taking a new drug and dealing with the side effects and putting up with the additional testing required by a clinical trial, she wouldn't have enough energy left to help her daughter make the plans for the pool and the surrounding garden. In the end, she said no to the clinical trial, knowing that it was the right decision for her.

What Is This Clinic I've Heard About Overseas?

Patients and families sometimes ask whether there are promising drugs in trials overseas, or they ask about experimental treatment regimens in other countries. One patient, for example, had a son who had read about a clinic in Mexico that claimed to be performing miracles with a nontraditional approach to treating cancer. They used a combination of Reiki therapy, massage therapy, shark cartilage, and nutritional cleanses that included coffee enemas to treat patients with cancer. It cost $30,000 for a one-week stay.

As doctors, we are often in a tough spot when patients want to pursue these kinds of treatments, and there are generally three major concerns. First, there is often no data showing these experimental approaches are effective in treating cancer. The second is that traveling to a small clinic in another country could be unsafe and make the patient's life very uncomfortable, and we also deeply worry that the patient could lose their life savings on these very expensive but otherwise unproven treatments.

In the end, though, we can only offer our opinions and worries. Patients and families make their own decisions. In this case, the son would not listen to the advice against the Mexico clinic, and the patient wanted to keep her family happy, so she agreed to fly to San Diego and then drive over the border. She took out a second mortgage on her condominium in Boston to pay cash for the treatment, as the clinic required. When she returned a little over a week later, she was dehydrated, plagued with diarrhea, and ten pounds lighter. It took three days to rehydrate her before it was safe to release her from the hospital and into hospice care. Her cancer had not responded at all to these treatments.

Patients can be under enormous pressure from their families to keep fighting using any available experimental treatments. Doctors often think about how to help patients and families see that there is more to this whole cancer experience than just living longer. It is about living *well*. For some patients it is about living longer at all costs, and for those patients no amount of suffering seems like too much. As doctors, this is difficult to watch. It just feels wrong to cause harm, and we don't feel comfortable prescribing treatments that will make people worse.

But I Can Still Beat This, Right?

When people are pushing hard to do more chemotherapy or try experimental treatments, there is often something at work behind this demand. Doctors sometimes refer to this as the tyranny of positive thinking. Some people tell themselves that if they can believe in and visualize a different future for themselves, they can change their own biology. Some people tell themselves that they can stop their cancer cells from growing if they have the right attitude. When patients or family members say this to us, we get worried.

In general, we would never discount the power of positive thinking. Cancer patients and their families go through so much in treatment, and many of them do it with such grace and strength—even humor—that we feel lucky to know them. We know they aren't battling the cancer itself but rather fighting to have as much of a normal life as they can despite this terribly unfair diagnosis and despite difficult treatment regimens. They have needed to stay positive and to believe in themselves to do all of that, and it's hard to express how much we admire this fortitude.

And yet we worry about people who say they know they will be cured if they just keep believing that as true. We've had crying patients tell us their cancer has grown because they didn't stay positive enough. Family members, too, have scolded us, saying the patient has to believe that they will be cured in order to be cured. "You aren't going to tell Mom that this is incurable, are you? You aren't going to tell her that she might die?" We've been asked some version of these questions many times. These scenarios break our hearts because it's not true. You can't wish cancer away.

Hope is an essential part of being human, of course, and we would never tell anyone to give up hope. We hope, too, that every patient will be the exception. We just want patients and family members to hold onto hope while still being able to understand the medical facts and to understand something about how the disease is likely to progress. This gives patients the chance to focus on the task of finding ways to live well.

By having this understanding, patients and family members can also make better decisions about what kind of treatments they want and don't want. For example, if chemotherapy brings a 70% chance of cure for a patient's breast cancer, that patient may choose to undergo this arduous treatment knowing that it has a real likelihood of allowing a good quality of life for years or decades afterward. When we say that a certain drug has a less than 10% chance of shrinking a tumor that we know won't ever be cured, or if it will likely extend life by only a couple of weeks, the patient might reasonably choose not to try it. We need to give our patients a realistic framework for understanding their illness and their treatment options. This is the heart of informed consent.

What Would You Advise Your Mother or Father to Do in This Situation?

Oncologists hear this question a lot from patients. Some of them hate to have to answer it, but Dave loves this question. The answer is incredibly valuable to patients as they navigate the difficult choices they have to make, and it's no different from asking a lawyer or an accountant or any other expert what they would do in your situation. Dave generally frames his answer by describing his parents. His mother is a devoutly religious woman who raised seven children. She hates the idea of chemotherapy and would never agree to it just to live a couple of extra months. She has said that if the good Lord wants her to live longer, he is in charge of that. Dave's father, on the contrary, was a bit of a risk taker. He might have taken a chance on a new experimental clinical trial that offered the possibility of a sustained response. What Dave hopes to explain to patients by talking about his parents is that there are no correct answers, only correct answers for you. The best way to make the right decision is to know what kind of person you are and how you want to live.

For every patient with metastatic breast cancer, there will come a point when stopping cancer treatments is the right thing to do. Supportive care and helping patients to feel as well as they can become the focus of good care. It may be easier to focus on chemotherapy rather than on the business of living. It's certainly easier for the oncologist, who can talk about abstract issues such as response rates and overall survival. But we want patients to focus more on what they want to do with the time they have left.

CHAPTER TWENTY-THREE

My Body Feels Like It's Shutting Down

As people start to feel more fatigued and spend more time in bed during the day, they wonder what the process of dying from breast cancer is like. How is it going to feel? Am I going to know when it's happening? Does it take a long time? In this chapter, we describe the possible outcomes as cancer continues to progress.

This is not an easy subject to think about or read about. People who aren't dealing with cancer often want to avoid thinking or talking about death, but so often patients do want to know how they will be taken care of and kept comfortable during the time when their bodies are shutting down. Some people take great comfort in knowing what might happen next and how diligently the hospice team, the oncology team, and the palliative care team will be working to help them at this time.

The first thing to know is that for most people with cancer, dying can be peaceful. Most people decline gradually and die in their sleep, and this is true even if they die of liver failure or infection. As people get closer to death, the hospice team can help patients and their families know what to expect and explain the many ways to help minimize discomfort or distress, even in the final hours of life. Of course, there are some instances where patients have an acute change in status, where they go from feeling relatively stable to needing hospitalization or admission to an inpatient hospice facility to get the kind of medical care that wouldn't be possible at home.

If you are hoping to stay home during this time, you'll need a lot of support from family and friends, and we'll describe why. At the same time, you may be wondering how to manage information that goes out to extended family and friends or how many people you want visiting you at this time. We can talk about ways that other people have handled these issues, but we also remind patients that they aren't dying yet. We've worked with people who have been in hospice care for a couple of months who say, "I can't believe that I'm still here." It can be tricky to figure out how to keep setting goals and keep finding things to look forward to, but you can do this.

Lastly, for many people, spiritual issues become more pronounced during this time, even for those who are not sure they believe in God or an afterlife. Hospitals have chaplains or a chaplaincy service that can help people talk through any spiritual questions that they may have.

How Will I Die?

Throughout this book, we've said that your medical team members may not be able to give you an exact time frame for how long you will live. But your oncologist should be able to tell you whether you are in the last six months of life. For most types of cancer, doctors know on average how long people live after each stage of treatment. This is a good time to ask your oncologist to give an approximate time frame for death because having some idea of whether you might live a few weeks, a few months, or more than six months can help you think about how you want to live during that time.

You can also ask your oncologist how you might die. A few oncologists may not like to hear these questions and may dismiss them because this is hard to talk about. Many oncologists, though, welcome these questions and any chance to talk to you about your wishes during the final phase of your life. People are sometimes worried about asking these questions and hearing the answers, but then they find the conversation actually eases their fears and helps them to make relevant decisions and have important conversations with their loved ones.

Typically, death comes by one of several pathways. It can be either a slow decline caused by the cancer or a more sudden acute process caused either by the cancer or by treatment.

The Slow Decline

The most common way people die from cancer is in a decline that occurs over many months. The patient becomes gradually more fatigued and spends more of the day in bed or asleep and begins to lose interest in eating. Although there may be pain or nausea or other symptoms, these are dependent on the location of any tumors and aren't universal.

The goal of the medical team is still to help you have a good quality of life, which means to be alert and comfortable. Sometimes your doctor may want to give medications to control symptoms even though they cause sedation. If the symptoms are difficult to control, you may need to trade comfort for alertness, but your doctor should ask you what you want. Do you want to be more alert to interact with family, or do you really want the pain to be minimized? Continuing to communicate your goals is paramount.

April was a 72-year-old woman with breast cancer who had had a terrific response with hormonal therapy for the first four years of treatment. Over the next couple of years, when the first therapy stopped working, she tried other hormonal therapies that were less successful. In her seventh year of treatment, she knew that her pain and fatigue were getting worse and she was losing weight, no matter what she ate. Her doctor tried several rounds of chemotherapy, but they didn't control the tumors. Eventually, she lost her appetite as well and knew that she was near the end of effective treatment.

April didn't want to disappoint her oncologist, who had been treating her from the beginning, so she asked her palliative care specialist what dying would be like and when it might occur. She was an immensely practical person who had lost her husband several years earlier, and so she knew what she needed to do to get her estate in order and signed an advance health directive and even made plans to travel while she could. Then she told her oncologist that she was done with chemotherapy and not interested in a clinical trial. She wanted to be enrolled in hospice, where she became quite friendly with her hospice nurse. For the next couple of months, she still came in to see the oncologist every two weeks and had her medications adjusted when she had new symptoms. She told her medical team that she was at peace with what was happening.

Gradually, April became more fatigued and had to miss an appointment. After that, it became clear that she needed help around the clock, because she had trouble getting to the bathroom on her own. Her children began taking turns sleeping at her house. Soon, she informed them that she wanted inpatient hospice care, which her nurse helped arrange for her. The next day an ambulance picked her up, and she moved with two suitcases to the hospice facility. She was soon bedbound and reported that she couldn't believe how fatigued she was. The hospice facility managed her pain and kept her comfortable, and in the third week she drifted into a coma and died 48 hours later with her family present.

During a slow decline, patients have time to take care of practical and personal matters. They see the cancer getting worse in multiple ways and gradually accept the prognosis (the likely course and outcome of their disease) and the inevitability of death. April was lucky to have both an oncologist and a palliative care physician with whom she could speak about her wishes. And she was lucky to have a supportive family, people who were available to stay with her when she needed help. April was also lucky in that she had a great awareness of her prognosis. During each step along the way she understood what the goals of treatment were and how they interacted with her overall goals of care. So she was able to choose an inpatient hospice facility when she didn't want her family members to feel that they had to bear sole responsibility for caring for her.

While we hope every patient has such a comfortable and gentle death, complications from cancer and treatment can occur at any step and turn a chronic process into an acute or subacute process. And when patients and families can acknowledge that dying is a possibility, we find it allows a more open dialogue that allows everyone to plan. People are sometimes afraid to think about death because they don't want other people to think that they are giving up. Sometimes they don't want the oncologist to think that they're giving up. Acknowledging the possibility of death is not equivalent to giving up, though. In all our years of caring for patients who are dying from cancer, we have rarely had anyone who didn't want more time even as they accepted the possibility of dying.

The Subacute Decline

Subacute decline is a medical event that can occur when patients have already begun to experience fatigue and other symptoms of advancing cancer. Patients can go from feeling relatively stable to being close to death over the course of a few weeks or days. It's less common than the slow decline, but patients should be aware that it can happen. Breast cancer can be a slow plodding course for many years and then metastatic lesions in places like the liver or the lining around the brain can cause a more rapid decline.

For years, Rita had a slow-growing metastatic breast cancer that came under control every time she tried chemotherapy. The chemotherapy would effectively manage the tumor growth for many months. One treatment even kept the growth at bay for over a year. Within a few weeks of starting any new therapy, she would feel better and her symptoms would greatly improve. Her treatment went on like this for several years, until one day she was overcome with fatigue. She looked in the mirror and noticed that the white part of her eyes looked a little bit yellow. Her oncologist took some scans and found that her previously indolent cancer in her bones and liver had, unfortunately, changed rapidly. Rita now, suddenly, had a liver that was nearly completely replaced with tumor.

Rita's liver was so damaged by the tumor that it was not safe to give her chemotherapy, and she lived with it not functioning well for several weeks. One day, though, Rita became confused and her family called the oncology team. Her oncologist took more scans and confirmed that her liver and kidneys were on the verge of shutting down. Her doctor stabilized her, made her comfortable, and then sent her home with hospice care and the support of her family. She died within 10 days of leaving the hospital.

Rita was fortunate that she had several years of slow-growing cancer, and she and her family knew that at some point the cancer would not be controlled by treatment anymore. Still, the sudden change in her condition was something they struggled to cope with. When treatments have been effective to control the cancer for long periods of time, this dramatic change in circumstances can be difficult to understand. In these cases of subacute decline, it is important to keep communicating with your medical team about what is happening, what treatment options are available, and how your plan for dying at home may need to give way to a plan B in which you get medical support during the final days if necessary.

Even if your doctor told you that you could hope for an additional 6 to 12 months of a gradual decline, that may not be possible if the cancer begins to move more aggressively or if a truly acute event happens. In these cases, communication among family members is crucial. Without it, some family members can panic and begin to argue over the next steps in treatment for the patient. There is always uncertainty in cancer treatment, which is why palliative care works with people to have important conversations about end-of-life care—it can become relevant without warning.

The Acute Decline

Occasionally a patient with cancer can develop a life-threatening condition within a few hours and without much warning. Thankfully, this is uncommon. These acute problems can stem from either the cancer or the treatment, and they can trigger a hospitalization and initiate the process of dying.

Acute events may result from clotting issues or rapid disease progression. A patient can have a blood clot go to the lungs or brain. Other times, an acute event may involve the worsening of liver function, deterioration in breathing because of progressive lung metastases, or fluid buildup around the lungs. While these events can occur at any time during cancer treatment, they are more likely to happen after the treatments have stopped working.

Jenn had a patient named Donna who had lived with metastatic breast cancer for six years and had been through several lines of therapy. Donna knew that her cancer was progressing, and she had been wondering about the possibility of enrolling in home hospice or starting a clinical trial. Donna had asked about her best-case scenario, and Jenn had told her that there were a couple more lines of chemotherapy that could be tried but that Jenn was worried that they would likely not be as effective as the previous treatments.

One day, Donna experienced sudden, severe chest pain and difficulty breathing. Donna's husband brought her to the emergency room, and doctors found that a massive blood clot had traveled from her pelvis to her lungs before dividing into multiple smaller clots. It was clear that her lungs and heart were already starting to shut down. Jenn had tried before to talk to her and her husband about her wishes for end-of-life care, but they had put these discussions off. Now Donna told Jenn that she didn't want to die in the intensive care unit. She knew that even if she had a breathing tube inserted, she was unlikely to ever leave the hospital and would probably never come off the ventilator. Donna decided that she wanted comfort management alone, which meant that she would receive morphine and other medications to ease the work of breathing.

Donna was admitted to a private room in the hospital where her family could be alone with her. Soon, she drifted off to sleep but could still be aroused by questions from her family. She could nod or shake her head to questions and smile at her family. Over the next few hours, her breathing pattern changed and became irregular. Doctors call this Cheyne-Stokes, which is a breathing pattern of slow, deep breaths followed by shallow, quick breaths. It's common as patients approach death but doesn't signal any distress or pain. Donna looked peaceful, and nurses continued to check on her to adjust her medications. Donna died comfortably later that evening surrounded by her family.

Women who have brain metastases can have acute neurologic events, in which tumor growth or new lesions in the lining around the brain can render them confused and disoriented. Brain metastases (tumors spread to the brain) can sometimes cause seizures as well. If this happens, doctors usually admit the patient to the hospital because it is difficult for families to manage these situations at home. Even if this happens, the medical team will work to keep the patient comfortable and help family members understand what's happening.

Help at Home

As the cancer advances and therapies become less effective, fatigue will become much more pronounced. At this point, doctors recommend home hospice care, which is a medical benefit that allows you to get extra care in your home. Most insurance policies cover this care. To qualify for home hospice, two doctors have to certify that they believe you have a prognosis of less than six months. Even if the doctors are wrong, though, and you live longer than six months, you won't be kicked out of hospice. Many people think that hospice care is for people who are actively dying, but that's not true. This crucial benefit can help you when you may have months to live.

Hospice does not provide 24-hour care in the home; rather, it allows for home visits from a nurse, and it allows you to get medications delivered to your home. You are required to have a weekly visit from a nurse, but you can have visits more often if needed, and most hospice providers offer a team, including social workers, who can offer emotional support to you and your family. There are chaplains who can visit you at home if you don't feel well enough to attend services. Home health aides can come to your house three to five days a week for a couple of hours at a time to help with daily living tasks. Many hospice services also engage volunteers who can spend time with you while a loved one runs an errand.

We usually suggest that people start with some home health aide help. This allows you to get used to someone coming to your house while you can still care for yourself. You can teach the home health aide how to best assist you, and you can figure out whether they are a good fit for you. Also, most people don't know how much their loved ones worry about leaving them alone. Family members sometimes don't confess their fears to the patient and end up feeling trapped in the house. Having a home health aide stop by for an hour or two can free them to do errands and take a break.

Even if you have engaged home hospice, you might need more support than you think you do. We often suggest making a plan to have friends and family in the home around the clock. If you've lived alone, this might be a good time to have family members stay in the house or to stay at a friend or family member's home. Your health status can change abruptly, but it will also change gradually, and you don't know when you might begin to have more trouble getting to the bathroom, staying hydrated, or even getting in and out of bed.

Eating and Drinking

As their bodies are slowing down due to advancing cancer, many patients don't have much interest in eating. Doctors don't worry at this stage about whether the patient is eating, but it can become a real battle with family members as loved ones insist that eating is important to keep up a patient's strength. But you don't have to eat or drink to please anyone, and it's not going to keep up your strength. In some cases, trying to eat when you don't feel like it can actually make you feel sick. Your body is giving you signals that it doesn't need much food or that it can't process food in the way it did before.

Doctors also don't recommend appetite stimulants at this point, and there is usually no reason to give extra fluids through an IV. When your body is slowing down, IV fluids can make you feel miserable, and sometimes the fluid pools in the stomach or lungs in a way that would require a procedure to drain it. This is the time to listen to your body's natural signals.

You Aren't Dying Yet

We often have to remind patients, even as they come to accept the possibility of dying, that they are actually still living with cancer. The role of palliative care is to help people live as well as they can, even when their bodies are slowing down and cancer treatments have stopped. There will come a time when you are in the last days or hours of life, but that hasn't happened yet. You still want to work to make sure that your symptoms are well treated. You may feel limited in your choice of activities, but you are still living and setting goals about how you want to spend your final weeks in ways that allow you to grow and think and connect with others.

I (Vicki) witnessed my patient Bonnie become a master at this. She found a variety of things she could do depending on her energy level. Some days she listed to podcasts of interesting topics or stories, such as *The Moth Radio Hour* or *This American Life*. Some days she felt up to reading. She and her daughters had read novels together throughout her illness. Their book group gave them something to talk about other than the illness and the uncertain future. This last phase of her life was no different. On days when she felt really crummy, she had videos cued up to watch that made her laugh or about topics that were interesting to her. Her friends and family kept her engaged and learning even in this final phase of her life. Another patient, Jenny, binged on every season of *Breaking Bad* in the last eight weeks of her life. She was hooked on that show, and it gave her something to distract herself and also to chatter with others about.

My patient Gail had been living for a long time with breast cancer when she got to this point. At 65, she had an extended family with grown kids and growing grandchildren. She knew that she wanted to be with her family as much as possible and to be somewhere outside. She wanted to be as active as possible when she felt good enough. At the same time, she had physical symptoms that needed medical attention. She had fluid building in her abdomen that needed to be drained every day. So we connected her with a hospice facility near her home. She had a large back porch and spent most of her time outside where she held court with family and friends and enjoyed the birds and the summer sun. She had a great time, resting when she needed, and eating a little bit when she felt able. On some days she was awake more, and on some days she slept or rested for much of the day. One day when she felt particularly strong, she attended her granddaughter's softball game and cheered from her wheelchair.

Gail also had a medical plan in place in case she needed acute medical care, even if she didn't want to die in the hospital. She knew that she could be admitted to a hospital with an inpatient hospice facility. Gail found a way to stay connected and to make choices that were meaningful to her about how to spend this time. This phase is sort of a marathon, not a sprint. Your doctors don't know how it is going to play out exactly, and there are still going to be good days for you.

For many people, spending time with friends and family feels critically important, and yet they worry about people sitting in some sort of vigil. They ask whether it's okay to laugh and whether it's okay just to be together without talking much. Of course it is. You can still forget about the illness and concentrate on spending time together.

One patient asked her grown children to lug all the photo boxes out of the attic so they could go through them together. Sarah had just a couple of hours each day when she felt energetic, but they would spend that time looking at photos and retelling the old stories behind them. On the days that she didn't feel up to this, she would watch classic movies that she and her family loved. It reminded them of all the lovely times they had shared together over the years.

The key is to find the balance between pushing yourself to engage in the world and resting when you need to. On days when you feel like you can swing it, get up and come into the world. Make plans for how you are going to spend the day. Maybe it is reading or visiting with a friend. These goals are probably quite different from the goals that you had when you were well, but it is vital to have them.

Communicating with Others

We've talked about how to communicate with extended family and friends about your illness at the time of diagnosis in the first chapters of the book and in chapter 21 as you start dealing with progressing cancer and potentially ending treatment. The same rules apply here. Your A orbit consists of those people who are closest to you, the people who have offered the most help and support at home and those who bring energy and joy into your life. These folks probably already know most of the details of your situation. People in your B or C orbits know potentially less about your prognosis, if anything at all. They love you, and many of them want to know more about how to help and how to offer support to your family. They might even want to send notes or call or visit, but they don't know what's okay and what would be intrusive. It can be helpful to find a way to communicate some details about how you are doing and guidelines about how these outer orbits can help or communicate with you if they want.

Some people choose to write a group email or post a message on a private website such as CaringBridge, which they can update as circumstances change. Someone in your A orbit can write these or simply be assigned to send out a message that you write. Be sure to think about how you want people to be in touch and state whether you want to have visitors and when those visits would be welcome. Seeing old friends and extended family can sometimes feed your energy level, but it can also deplete your energy. Or, as one patient once said, "So many people want to come and see me before I die. It's nice." And then she added dryly, "My nephew's fiancé, though, I could have done without that one." Even if you aren't up to a lot of visitors, people might be encouraged to send notes or emails sharing their memories and good wishes that you can read on your own time.

I've included here a letter that a patient of mine wrote to his family and gave me permission to share. Although Alexander wasn't a breast cancer patient, I love this letter because he is so open about what's happening and yet he is clear about the love and gratitude that he has for his life and for the people who will be reading the letter. Alexander told me that after he sent it, he received the most powerful response from his extended network of friends. People were deeply touched by the letter, and many wrote to him to say so. You don't have to write a letter like this, but it can be useful to see how others have handled this type of communication.

Dear Friends,

I sit here at dusk, looking out of a genuinely lovely room at MGH, and think of how deeply fortunate I am to have you all, my wife Lisa, my boys, my home, the beauty of this sunset over the Charles, and the many relationships and experiences that have made my life as rich and wonderful as it is. I am happy with my life and have lived well, without regret.

As many of you know, my year-and-a-half battle with this uncommon gastrointestinal cancer has had its ups and downs, during which I have received extraordinary care from MGH and, as needed, Dana-Farber Cancer Institute. Through October I had been coping with the gradual spread of the cancer reasonably enough. However, last Wednesday I had a PET scan (nuclear medicine that highlights locations of likely cancerous activity) and a CT scan (more detailed imaging of bone, muscle, and tissue) that displayed a thoroughly new picture of my body. Unfortunately, Wednesday's scans showed an aggressive spread into my hips, back, pelvis, lungs, and brain, with several ribs fractured due to the disease and a blood clot in a lung, which whisked me back into the hospital for immediate attention and monitoring.

And so I have turned the corner into my last chapter. We have known this was coming—my cancer was identified some time ago as uncurable—but we did not expect as sudden a shift as this. So we will accommodate it, as we have each setback along the way that this cancer has presented. The surprise was for my boys, William, sixteen, and Andrew, thirteen. We told them on Saturday afternoon in perhaps the toughest moment our family has ever had. They have always known the uncurable aspect of my cancer and were aware all treatments had failed, but we had not previously introduced the soon-to-be-fatal feature of my cancer—out of respect to let them live their teenage lives without the cloud of my imminent death constantly over their heads. They also were not fully aware my demise would be so soon: months, not years. I now have probably two to six weeks to live; my doctors still find it difficult to identify and forecast how the spreading cancer will bring my days to an end.

My boys are strong and courageous, and Lisa is a rock. Our afternoon meeting was traumatic, and it was but the start of a long process to absorb loss and grief and again move forward. I have full faith that the three of them will find a path back to happiness, however they construct that, and find a way to celebrate my memory, feel my ongoing love, and know that their lives hold plenty of joy, challenge, beauty, and satisfaction across the years ahead.

I expect to be discharged from MGH today, after some further radiation to kill pockets of cancer in my hips and back, where it could still do painful damage in a short time. I will also return for specialized radiation that aims to kill the two small tumors in my brain, which could also cause trouble if untreated. My discharge will be to hospice care at home, which has long been our plan, and I will stay at home so long as it works well for all. If I need to be in a facility, I will enter a lovely one in Danvers, Massachusetts, that is the inpatient location for the at-home hospice organization Care Dimensions.

My energy is low, and some days I get only three to four really good hours in the morning and then a drowsy afternoon and evening focused on pain management, as the evenings and overnights are usually my most challenging. I would love to see so many of you as your own schedules permit, and maybe that will work for us in many instances. But I do tire easily, and I have yet to see what my decline over this period at home or in Danvers will be like, so I'm keeping my expectations modest. I always value and appreciate an email, a card, or a poem; and phone calls are good but too can be tiring, depending on how the day is going.

I am so grateful for the support, care, and love you have shown me. I am sorry my life has to end now and curtail the relationships that have made, and continue to make, my existence the rich, fun, exciting, and worthy journey it's been. There are silver linings everywhere, if you know to look for them, and I have grown immensely in the past nineteen months. I wouldn't wish this experience, or this premature death, on anybody, but some of the new closeness, deepened relationships, revelations of character, and demonstrations of love I have received have left me moist-eyed at what my friends have done for me and what good people will do for each other.

Thank you. It is a genuine pleasure to have spent the time we have. Stay well. Please reach out to my wife and boys over the months and years after I'm gone. And when you do, remember me with a smile.

Yours,
Alexander

CHAPTER TWENTY-FOUR

What Is a Good Death?

Many people tell us that they want a good death. And for most people Vicki, Jenn, and I have worked with, a good death means they hope to be free of pain or other discomfort and to be surrounded by the people they love. They also hope to have achieved some acceptance about their own death. Not everyone who is facing death feels at peace, though. Others feel that there is no way death can be good. We wish a good death was possible all the time, but everyone has a different idea of what that means or if it is even possible.

As difficult as it might be to think about and talk about death, we find that articulating what you want at the end of life helps many patients feel more in control. Some people do want to be at home during their final days and hours, and others consider having daily physical care being done by family unthinkable because they don't want their immediate family to feel burdened or stressed. It's important for families to hear the patient's wishes, even if not every wish can be carried out. How someone dies is part of how they lived. The person who is dying should have some say in what happens and where it happens.

In this chapter, I outline some of the issues that people should think about when having these conversations about how to have this final phase of life go as well as possible.

Dying at Home

I worked with a patient early in my career who had metastatic breast cancer that had spread to her liver. Monica was 79 years old and had an extended family that included her husband, five children, and 17 grandchildren. She also had several siblings with large families. Her grandchildren were old enough to take turns sleeping in a cot next to Monica's bed so they could help her get to the bathroom in the middle of the night. Her last days were spent playing cards or having people read to her. In the rest of the house, people gathered after work or school to share stories. Walking into that house always made me happy, because it was filled with love and kindness. I remember saying to Monica that I hoped my death would be like this, in a home filled with people laughing and talking. Monica had minimal pain and greeted everyone with a smile. Gradually she lost energy and drifted into a coma that lasted for about 12 hours before she died peacefully in her sleep.

Monica was lucky in several ways. First, her symptoms were easy to control. She didn't suffer from delirium or confusion, and she didn't have a lot of pain or dizziness or shortness of breath. Second, she had an extended family of healthy adults who wanted to care for her. Her grandchildren had extra time and energy to help by spending the night with her and taking care of her daily tasks, including helping her to the bathroom, helping her wash herself, changing her sheets, and getting whatever bites of food she felt able to eat. Third, Monica and her family understood that she was dying and that the purpose of treatment was to keep her comfortable. If you took away one or two of these factors, dying at home would not have been possible for Monica or any other patient.

Palliative care clinicians ask specific questions of patients who say they want to die at home. No one wants a patient to go home to a situation that's untenable for the family or one that isn't safe. If you are in a hospital and want to be discharged to your home to die, your medical team will want to talk about several factors.

Have you enrolled in hospice care? It is essential to have medical professionals involved who are experts in end-of-life care. In addition, you may need to hire additional home health aides, and if so, you'll want to know what the cost would be.

Are your symptoms well controlled? Your doctor will want to be reassured that your pain is under control with medication and that you are medically stable enough to leave the hospital. No one wants your family to suffer at home through a medical crisis in which your symptoms flair and you become distressed. We have learned to pay attention to the level of anxiety patients express about going home. In other words, patients often know when their home situation will likely be overwhelming. The goal is to make sure you can die at home while staying peaceful and comfortable.

How much help is available at home? You need adults staying with you in the house who can help with washing, toileting, and preparing any food. Hospices require that patients have someone with them at all times. What most people don't realize about hospice is that it is not 24-hour care. The lion's share of the care falls to family caregivers. Providing this kind of care for a loved one is hard, and it works best if there are several people to take turns staying with you, and you might need two people inside the house at all times. That sounds like a lot of help, and it is, but it's a good benchmark to make sure that there are enough adults around who can give breaks to immediate family members. Otherwise, it is just too hard to provide the appropriate care. This is why dying at home doesn't work for everyone.

Are there any other issues that would make home care difficult? If a patient is struggling with confusion or delirium or if they are not able to stand because of dizziness or unable to cross the room even with assistance because of shortness of breath, a doctor might wonder whether dying at home is still possible. One palliative care clinician we know cared for her mother-in-law at home while she was in the advanced stages of pancreatic cancer. Although the mother-in-law was an independent woman who was able to care for herself throughout her illness, in the end she struggled with balance issues from brain metastases. This became worse as her liver function declined and her body wasn't able to metabolize medication easily. She developed worsening confusion and fell several times. Our colleague is a medical professional in palliative care who truly wanted to help her loved one and care for her in a home setting, but in this case the best option for the patient was a residential treatment facility where she could get the care she needed.

Dying at a Residential Hospice

Sometimes family isn't nearby or a patient doesn't feel comfortable having loved ones take on the burden of care. Sometimes the illness doesn't allow for patients to die at home.

If dying at home isn't possible, some people choose a residential hospice. Think of this as a setting that feels more like home than a hospital. In a residential hospice, nurses and aides can care for you 24 hours a day. It's not the same intensity of care as you will find in a hospital, but there are nurses and aides available all the time.

Tonya is a patient who had been treated for metastatic breast cancer for several years. She enrolled in hospice and planned to spend her remaining time at home with her three teenagers. Her kids were enthusiastic about this idea, and Tonya's sister moved back to Boston to be near her and help her out. A few weeks later, it became clear to everyone that this was not going to work out the way they'd hoped. As her fatigue worsened, Tonya found that she needed help around the clock, including help to get to the bathroom in the middle of the night. Her kids were showing signs of stress, and one of them had become angry and withdrawn. Tonya realized that she wanted her house to be a safe place for her kids after she died, and she feared that these memories would make that impossible. She decided to enroll in a residential hospice for the last few weeks of her life.

In most cases, families need to pay a daily rate at a residential hospice facility. It is usually a sliding scale between $200 and $500 a day. In Tonya's case, a palliative care specialist helped to petition her health insurer to pay this daily fee because the residential hospice offered better and less expensive care than she would receive in a nursing home. I spoke to Tonya's sister shortly after she died, and she confirmed that this was the right decision. The kids came to see her every day and they could spend as much time as they wanted, sometimes staying for whole days on the weekends. They were able to see her as their mother rather than a patient, which is what she wanted. Those last weeks were spent looking at old photographs, telling stories, and just hanging out.

Dying in an Inpatient Hospice

For some patients, dying in a hospital setting might be the best choice. When patients have symptoms that are difficult to control—such as nausea, confusion, or pain—the intensive treatment available at the hospital may be the best approach to keep them comfortable and free of distress.

Jenn had a patient named Sally, a music teacher, who had been treated for a particularly aggressive triple-negative breast cancer. It had grown through all of the chemotherapy treatments and eventually spread to her brain. Sally went through two weeks of radiation therapy to control these brain lesions. Although the treatments worked, they left her exhausted and unsure of herself. Sometimes she woke up in the middle of the night with pain but didn't feel confident that she was taking the right medications. Sally had no immediate family living nearby. Her elderly parents lived in another state and had their own health issues. She asked her friends for help but felt overwhelmed by her own situation. Sally would probably have been a good candidate for residential hospice, but then her pain became harder to control. Eventually, she needed IV pain medication to stay comfortable.

In the last weeks of her life, Sally moved into a nice inpatient hospice facility paid for by her insurance. The staff was able to adjust her pain medications frequently so she didn't have to worry about pain or which medications to take. Her friends and many former students came by to talk with her and share memories and concert videos. Her parents also visited every day, and she died peacefully in her sleep.

Dying in the Intensive Care Unit

Vicki, Jenn, and I spend a lot of time talking to patients who have advanced cancer about preparing for the possibility of death, taking care of practical matters, and thinking about where they would like to be when they die. We do this because we hope patients can form a plan for what to do if the cancer gets worse. We also do it because we want patients to avoid dying in the intensive care unit (ICU) if possible.

All cancer specialists and palliative care specialists have worked with patients who refuse to think about death and refuse to make any plan for it. And by the time the cancer progresses to the point that it is affecting multiple systems in their bodies—their liver and kidney function, their bowels, their lungs—they don't have options for the kind of medical care that would allow them to die peacefully with family and friends nearby. When a medical crisis arises, they may find themselves admitted to a hospital ICU, where they receive intensive treatments that are uncomfortable, even painful, and distressing for their families. And none of these intensive end-of-life treatments do anything to modify the cancer that caused the crisis.

Death in the ICU is often traumatic for all involved. Doctors recommend medical interventions that have a good chance of helping the patient to feel better and to live longer, if possible. These include medications to minimize discomfort or treat infection. Unfortunately, if someone is dying from cancer, putting that person on a breathing machine (ventilator) or performing CPR (resuscitation) will not improve quality of life. For the vast majority of people dying from complications of advanced cancer, these interventions will not bring a person back to life. In these situations, such intensive measures as a ventilator and CPR do not work, and even if they do, they may extend life for only a short time. Additionally, families may have to make difficult decisions about discontinuing life support or other measures that are not medically helpful.

Doctors know that people want to live as fully as they can for as long as they can. But, when they are dying, they don't want that process to be prolonged or uncomfortable. So, when doctors see patients with metastatic cancer die in the ICU, we consider it a bad death because we know it could have been more peaceful.

What If I Don't Want to Prolong My Dying?

Of course, people want to live longer even when they are living with illness. And yet when they are in the last hours or days of life, most people don't want to prolong the experience of dying. To best serve the patient, medical professionals use an ethical principle called patient autonomy. It states that patients who are of sound mind, who are not confused or depressed, have the right to refuse treatments they don't want.

Many interventions can prolong the process of dying, and patients have the right to decline them. They may choose to stop supplemental nutrition and hydration, antibiotics treating an infection, or blood thinners. We've had patients say to us, "Why can't we turn off my pacemaker so that I can die of my heart problems instead of the cancer?" The answer is that doctors can do that, and it is often a comfortable way to die. Any patient has the right to refuse treatment even if that treatment is life sustaining or life prolonging.

Patients sometimes choose not to take antibiotics for pneumonia in the final days of life. They do this because dying from pneumonia or any other infection can be very peaceful. People get drowsy as their blood pressure drops and drift away while sleeping. It can feel odd to talk about the final phase of life like this, but many people become practical and clear-eyed about choosing a gentle death.

Some people don't have any medical interventions that they can refuse because they don't have a growing infection or heart condition, but they can still make the decision to stop eating and drinking. Many people with advanced cancer aren't particularly interested in eating already, and they just stop pushing themselves to take in food and fluids. They keep their mouths moist with swabs but don't track their fluid intake and eventually become sleepier. This is a painless and gentle choice to make.

What Is Physician Aid in Dying?

In some states, doctors are allowed to assist patients who are critically ill and want to end their lives. As of this writing, it is legal in California, Colorado, District of Columbia, Hawaii, Montana, Maine, New Jersey, New Mexico, Oregon, Washington, and Vermont. Each state has its own regulations, but they share several common features. In most states, the patient must be a resident of the state in which this is legal. More than one physician must certify that the patient has a terminal diagnosis and that the patient request is not made under duress or because of depression or untreated symptoms. Typically the medication used, which is usually a powerful barbiturate sedative, is prescribed only after a waiting period. Also, the patient must be able to take the medication without the assistance of another person.

The law in Oregon has been in effect since 1997, and we know that not all the patients who acquire the prescription actually use it. We also know that most who do use it are not doing so because of suffering from symptoms but because they want to have control over the timing of their deaths. Doctors have very mixed feelings about physician aid in dying. Some believe that it is a patient's right to make this decision, while for others it runs counter to every instinct they have about the role of medicine in our lives.

Will My Family Be Okay during This Last Phase?

Family members will need extra help in the last few days. This allows for primary caregivers to take breaks, which is critical. They need extra people available or stopping by frequently to make sure that they have food and can rest because it's easy to stop taking care of oneself when so focused on the patient. They may also need extra help staying on top of the details of their regular lives, someone to walk the dog, or a hand running errands.

Sometimes families and friends have a large group around all the time, which is called sitting vigil. This can be a joyful time, with people laughing and sharing stories. But it can also be hard because no one knows how long this final phase in someone's life will last. Vicki often tells patients and family members that this stage of the illness can be more like a marathon than a sprint. There is still tremendous uncertainty. Be aware that you can always ask questions of hospice nurses about how events might unfold day to day. Caregivers should take the time to eat, rest, go for walks, and pace themselves.

Some people ask whether it's okay to die at home when children are present. There isn't a lot of data to guide us on this. Doctors often recommend that the dying patient stay in a space that affords some privacy so they can have quiet when they need it and so that children can have space to play and be kids but can still interact with the person who is dying as much as they want to or need to.

The next few sections address your family members and other concerns they might have.

How Families Can Prepare

In the final days of life, people often experience new symptoms, including pain, shortness of breath or noisy breathing, and confusion. In the vast majority of cases, these can be well controlled with medication. If the patient isn't already on an opioid, they may need one at this time to manage pain and shortness of breath. Haloperidol can help with confusion and delirium. Lorazepam will help with anxiety. There are also medications to treat the noisy breathing in the last hours of life, including atropine or hyoscyamine. Hospice providers often send a package of medications, called a comfort care kit, which contains many of these medications.

Still, the job of any hospice care team is to actively manage symptoms in the home and to be the eyes and ears of the oncology team. Make sure to call the patient's hospice team if symptoms are not being well controlled. If the hospice can't control them at home, the patient can still be admitted to an inpatient hospice facility or hospital, with the idea that they can return home once the symptoms have been stabilized.

Family members sometimes ask whether they can give too much pain medication and accidentally kill a patient. As long as you are following the guidelines of the hospice nurse or a physician, everything should be fine. If you have concerns about the amount of pain medication to give, though, you should call the hospice nurse for guidance. Sometimes the medical team will give enough pain medication to make patients comfortable even if they are sleepy or groggy much of the time as a result.

The primary goal is to make sure that the patient continues to be comfortable and free of distress.

As people get closer to dying, their breathing pattern often becomes quite erratic with quick bursts of respirations interspersed between long, slow, deep breaths and sometimes with gaps in breathing of 20 seconds or more. This is called Cheyne-Stokes respiration, and it usually means that people are in their final hours to days of life. If this breathing pattern starts and a hospice nurse isn't present, then you should call the nurse, who will want to know. Sometimes the patient's breathing can sound coarse and noisy, but there is no need to panic. This is a normal part of the dying process. All human beings go through it. Vicki always tells the family to look at the person's face. If the brow looks furrowed or the person looks restless, then more medication may be needed to ease the breathing. If the person looks comfortable and the breathing is just noisy, then they are not suffering.

Family Unity

I grew up in a large extended family, and one of my uncles was a priest who worked as a hospital chaplain. Early in my career as an oncologist, I asked him what the most amazing thing he had learned in his work helping dying patients was. He told me that when people are dying, they become even more exaggerated forms of their true selves. What he meant was that if people are kind and gentle at heart, they become even more so as they are dying. If people are ornery at heart, they become even more so as they are dying. And, he said, the same is often true for the family who has to care for the dying patient. The stress of dying for both the patient and family is enormous, and family discord can lead to a bad death even if the symptoms are well controlled and there is a lot of extra help at home.

Vicki had a patient named Sylvia with advanced metastatic breast cancer. During her treatment, there were frequent family meetings that included Sylvia's husband and their two daughters, who were both in college at the time. These meetings were fraught with tension and bickering. Sylvia revealed to Vicki that her husband had left her and filed for divorce at the time of her diagnosis. He then changed his mind and came home, but the daughters couldn't forgive him. They challenged everything he suggested as their mother's patient advocate. Sylvia really wanted her daughters to reconcile with their father because she knew they would need him after she died. She also worried about dying at home if that meant her daughters would be reluctant to visit and help with her care.

Believe me, your medical team knows when members of a family are carrying out a long-standing feud or when family members are fighting and taking sides over treatment decisions. Nurses in particular have a sixth sense for this, and they worry about patients going home to die in an environment filled with friction.

Sometimes families can put their differences aside for the good of the patient. Other times, they can't, and this puts the patient at risk of having a bad death. In these cases, it is usually best for everyone if the care is delivered in a setting other than home.

Being Present at the Moment of Death

Family members also ask how to prepare for the moment of death. These questions come in lots of forms. Some ask whether the patient might be afraid to leave the family, or they wonder whether they need to offer reassurances that it's okay to go. Many dying patients can still hear what is said to them even when they are no longer responding. It can be helpful to continue to talk to the person who is dying as though they can hear you. I've heard Vicki encourage loved ones to say whatever they feel comfortable communicating to the patient. That might include reassurances that it will be okay if they go and that you love them.

Some family members do want to travel to sit vigil or to say good-bye as death approaches. If family members feel that they want to see the patient one last time, it's okay to encourage them to come and sit vigil. They should make plans knowing that they might not be able to be there at the moment of death. As an alternative, they can call and say what they have to say to the patient, even if the patient can't respond. Or they can compose a message that someone sitting with the patient can read aloud. The important thing is for individuals to be able to communicate what they want to your loved one.

Some people want to be present at the moment of their loved one's death. While the idea of being present at death can seem significant, it's not always possible. Many times, I've seen patients hang on and die only after some significant family member arrives to see them. It's as though they were waiting. And these stories are the ones that get repeated to friends. But patients don't or can't always wait for family members to arrive. They also sometimes die while family members are using the bathroom or out getting coffee or sleeping. What I've learned is that the person who is dying seems to do this in their own way, and none of us can control when the moment of death will arrive.

Vicki often tells the story of her mother's death in Wisconsin. Vicki flew out from Boston to be with her mother during her final hours, but the cab driver got lost on the way from the airport to the nursing facility. When Vicki told the driver that she was going to see her dying mother, the cab driver started talking about his wife, who had died six months before. The more he talked, the more flustered and lost he became. Eventually, she arrived at her mother's side just a few minutes after her death. Vicki says that while being with her mother again was important to her, she understood that nothing could negate the love that she had for her mother or all of the ways she had worked to show her love over the years.

How Do We Know That Someone Has Died?

Doctors look for several signs that indicate that the patient has died. First, we touch the patient and look for a response. Next, we observe the person's breathing. This is a bit tricky in patients in the final hours of life because there may be pauses of a minute between breaths at the very end. These are the signs most families look for at home. When a clinician comes to verify the death, he or she will listen with a stethoscope to make sure that there are no heart sounds and examine the patient's eyes. When people die, their pupils don't respond to light, and they become fixed in a dilated, or open, state.

If you are sitting with a loved one, you might first notice that they are not responding to you. And then you'll watch for a minute or so and see no breathing movements. Also, don't be surprised if the skin has turned pale and bluish in the extremities and becomes cold to the touch or if the patient has become incontinent of urine or stool. We tell families to expect that everything will relax as the person dies. When you notice these signs, the next step is to call your hospice nurse if they are not already at your home. The hospice nurse will verify that the person has died. Once the hospice nurse has verified the death, they will likely wash the person's body and remove any medical equipment, such as IVs or oxygen lines. Families can choose to be present for this care and even participate if they would like. That may sound strange, but some families find it a meaningful way to pay their final respects.

The nurse will then call either the patient's oncologist, palliative care physician, or hospice doctor to sign the death certificate. You can then call the funeral director, who will send someone to your home to remove your loved one on a stretcher. If someone dies and is not enrolled in hospice, an ambulance is required by law in many states to bring a patient to the hospital to be pronounced dead. That's one of the many reasons why doctors advise patients to enroll in hospice.

Bereavement

The hours and days immediately following a person's death are typically busy. Family members may have services to prepare for, and there are guests who come to pay their respects. This is an emotional time that can often pass in a blur. And then friends and more distant relatives go back to their regular lives. Loved ones tell us that this is the hardest part. They ask themselves, "What now?"

The bereavement period is always one of firsts. First meals without someone, the first holidays, the first family vacation, the first time you want to call the person only to realize you can't. These are hard. Some memories are comforting, while others are painful. Vicki often tells people that it's hard to know how you will feel at any given point in grieving. Sometimes your friends think you should be sad, and you will feel okay. Other times, your friends will think you should be getting back into the rhythm of your life, and instead you feel like you've been hit by a truck and all you can do is cry all day. These feelings are all normal. It's important to be kind to yourself throughout this process.

Sometimes you might need additional support during the grieving process. Every hospice offers bereavement support services. This might be in the form of support groups or individual short-term counseling. You can take part in these services even if your loved one wasn't enrolled in hospice. Any hospice that receives federal support is required to provide bereavement services to anyone in its area.

In the weeks and months that follow someone's death, you may find that you still have the opportunity to be in a relationship with the person who has died. It's a very different kind of relationship, but it's still there. Often families will tell me, "I know what Mom would think about this. It sounds crazy, but I still feel like I can have a conversation with her."

It's also normal to have questions for the clinical care team about the patients' care after they have died. Vicki, Jenn, and I, like most clinicians, are happy to talk to loved ones after the death of a patient. Sometimes we do this to answer questions, and sometimes it is just to check in and say a final good-bye. We always call the family after one of our patients has died. We know how hard families work to support a patient during cancer care. Often close family members need someone to talk to about what their loved one experienced during the final days and hours before death. Sometimes, a member of the clinical team is the only person with whom you feel you can share these details. Cancer treatment can bring doctors, nurses, patients, and families close together. We like the opportunity to check in as well and to express to family members what was special about their loved one.

Vicki, Jenn, and I hope that this book can be a resource and a comfort for patients at every stage of cancer. It is our hope that this book empowers readers to ask the necessary questions of their doctors and to engage with their care teams in a meaningful way. We also want to demonstrate what care can be like when oncology and palliative care work together, because these two disciplines together can do more for patients than either can do alone. As an oncologist working closely with Vicki and Jenn, I've learned that integrating palliative care and cancer treatment helps patients to better understand their diagnosis and to better manage their symptoms throughout treatment so that they can live as well as they can for as long as they can.

We feel honored to do this work, and we hope that has shone through in these pages. We get to witness the courage of patients and families as they endeavor to live fully despite an uncertain future. It is enormously rewarding and humbling to care for patients with cancer. We have learned so much from our patients, each of whom have been extraordinarily generous to us by sharing their insights but also by allowing us to see their strength, creativity, and humor while facing this difficult diagnosis. Vicki, Jenn, and I are better parents, spouses, and physicians because of our relationships with our patients. They have taught us everything we needed to know to write this book.

David P. Ryan, MD

BREAST CANCER RESOURCES FROM HOPKINS PRESS

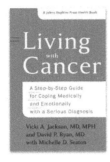

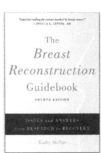

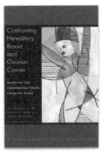

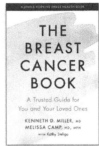

Living with Cancer

A Step-by-Step Guide for Coping Medically and Emotionally with a Serious Diagnosis

Vicki A. Jackson, MD, MPH, and David P. Ryan, MD, with Michelle D. Seaton

A comprehensive and compassionate guide for patients and families living with the physical and emotional effects of cancer.

Confronting Hereditary Breast and Ovarian Cancer

Identify Your Risk, Understand Your Options, Change Your Destiny

Sue Friedman, DVM, Rebecca Sutphen, MD, and Kathy Steligo foreword by Mark H. Greene, MD

"An insightful and informative read."
—*Nursing Times*

The Breast Reconstruction Guidebook

Issues and Answers from Research to Recovery, 4th ed.

Kathy Steglio

The definitive guide to breast reconstruction.

The Breast Cancer Book

A Trusted Guide for You and Your Loved Ones

Kenneth D. Miller, MD, and Melissa Camp, MD, MPH, with Kathy Steligo

A comprehensive, down-to-earth guide for anyone diagnosed with breast cancer.

press.jhu.edu

 @JHUPress

 @JohnsHopkinsUniversityPress

 @HopkinsPress

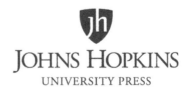